Disease
and
History

Disease
and
History

by

Frederick F. Cartwright

in collaboration
with Michael D. Biddiss

Rupert Hart-Davis   London

Granada Publishing Limited
First published 1972 by Rupert Hart-Davis Ltd
3 Upper James Street London W1R 4BP

ISBN 0 246 10537 2
Printed in Great Britain by
Northumberland Press Limited, Gateshead

WZ 40

Contents

Author's Preface

This book does not pretend to be an exhaustive account of the many ways in which disease has influenced the course of history. It is, in some measure, experimental for it became apparent quite early in the preparation of the manuscript that the subject could be covered only in a series of volumes. This has necessarily entailed selection and, all too often, the rejection of much interesting material. Tuberculosis, for instance, is of great historical importance but the effects have been too widespread to be linked with a single incident or person.

The ultimate decision whether to include or reject has been mine, and I must also accept full responsibility for the final text, but I am particularly fortunate in having enjoyed the collaboration of a professional historian. Dr Michael Biddiss, Fellow and Director of Studies in History at Downing College, Cambridge, has assiduously drawn my attention to sources of information, has discussed each chapter with me before and during the writing, and has read the final version. Not least of his services has been to restrain me when I, perhaps inevitably, have fallen into the error of overstressing the effect which disease has exerted upon a historical event.

I have also received much help from my friends. Mr Christopher Long spent many hours of library research during the early stages and provided me with a large amount of useful material, for which I am very grateful. As always, my colleagues at King's College Hospital have patiently answered my innumerable questions and generously given me the benefit of their specialized knowledge. Here I must particularly thank Dr D. W. Liddell, Dr C. G. McKerron, Dr S. Nevin and Dr Philip Hugh-Jones, who have read chapters and advised me upon the content. The Library Staff of King's College Hospital Medical School have, it is hardly necessary to add, been most generous with help and advice. Nor must I omit Mr Hugh Rawson of Thomas Y. Crowell Company, New York, and Mr Alan Brooke of Rupert Hart-Davis, London, who have not only criticized and edited the text but have supplied much information.

After some consideration it has been decided to omit references. But, of course, a great number of books have been consulted. The major debts are acknowledged in the bibliographical guide to further reading. This has been expanded to include works that deal with either the medical or the historical aspects of certain subjects more fully than the necessarily restricted space of the present volume will allow.

F. F. CARTWRIGHT.
Department of the History of Medicine,
King's College Hospital,
London, S.E.5.

Introduction

Historians and doctors have much in common. Both acknowledge that the proper study of mankind is Man. Both are
particularly interested in the influences which condition
human existence. The object of this book is to study the area
in which doctor and historian inevitably meet, that of the
impact of disease upon history. In medical diagnosis, a single
cause for disease will often be found. In historical investigation, the causes are likely to be complex. Nothing could be
more ridiculous than to contend that disease is always the
primary cause of a great historical change; but, particularly
at a time when the sociological aspects of history are being
emphasized, it is worth examining those episodes in which

the influence of disease may have been of real importance, especially when that importance has been neglected or misconstrued by more conventional historians.

Our aim in studying some of the various maladies which have afflicted the world will be to illustrate their effect not only upon historically important individuals, but also upon the peoples. Thus the study is relevant to History, whether conceived as a saga of great figures or as the story of social conditions and general human development. The ills that have plagued civilized man are as much a part of civilization as are their prevention and cure. If disease itself is historically important, then the conquest of disease is no less so. And, as we shall see, this conquest, though as yet only partial, has raised problems which are no less daunting for being different and which are just as relevant to our subject.

Man is a gregarious animal and the picture of primitive man isolated in his cave is misleading. The family unit soon developed into a tribe living a compact, communal life. Such small communities, which still exist in a few remote jungles today, dwelt in man-made clearings, with little or no contact between individual communities, for the high trackless forest prevented easy communication. Each community was self-supporting, dependent upon the plantain tree and cassava for its food. Bananas and manioc formed the staple diet, varied by small quantities of palm oil and only very rarely by flesh, either human or animal. The few enemies of these tribal communities were snakes, the occasional wild beast, pygmy tribes who shot at them with strophanthin-poisoned arrows. Puerperal fever in childbirth, a high infant mortality and endemic disease—malaria, sleeping sickness, yaws—prevented any rapid increase of population. Life span was short, for there was no known cure for any of the diseases from which these people suffered and a high carbohydrate diet led to early obesity with fatty infiltration of the vital organs. So tribal growth was almost static, increasing when live births outnumbered deaths, decreasing when infant mortality was high. Such is the slow natural process of increase in a community which is adequately fed and protected from major disaster, yet which is unable to cope with the hazards of childbirth and sickness.

Disaster in the form of famine, war, or epidemic disease could strike only from outside. A plague of insects might descend upon the crops and cause famine. Arab slavers, pushing down from the north and east of Africa, might chance upon one of these remote villages, engage the inhabitants in battle and carry off the survivors into captivity. In later years the white man would come, bringing with him new diseases, harmless enough to himself, but lethal to a community lacking inbred or acquired resistance.

Thousands of years ago man began to emerge from these primitive self-contained communities and the chances of major disaster multiplied. A greater degree of civilization brought benefits, a higher standard of living and a fuller, more intellectual life, but it also brought grave hazards. As more highly civilized peoples pushed out from their centres into less civilized districts, the chance of contact with unknown disease increased. Roads meant easier and faster travel and new diseases were able to pass more swiftly along such roads, striking down unprotected populations in mass pandemics before resistance to the invading organism could develop. City-dwelling people necessarily relied upon an extraneous food supply; if that supply failed there were no natural resources to take its place and famine became inevitable. Hunger, the desire for more and better living space, or the simple lust of a chieftain for power, would then set one tribe to fight against another. So man's three great enemies, Pestilence, Famine and War—the three Horsemen of the Apocalypse who bring in their train the Fourth Rider, Death upon his Pale Horse—developed on a larger scale.

Pestilence, famine and war interact and produce a sequence: war drives the farmer from his fields and destroys his crops; destruction of the crop spells famine; the starved and weakened populace fall easy victims to the onslaught of pestilence. All three are diseases. Pestilence is a disorder of man. Famine results from a disorder of plants and cattle, whether caused by abnormal weather or more directly by insect or bacterial invasion. War is a mass psychotic disorder. In this study, although the diseases of famine and war must necessarily have their place, our primary concern will be with those physical ills that have affected man directly.

I

Disease in the
Ancient World

Disease associated with civilization is older than written history, for civilization of a kind existed before the earliest records were kept. There is evidence of disease and of its sometimes important consequences at a comparatively early stage of recorded human development. The earliest known textbook of medicine, the *Great Herbal* of the Emperor Shen Lung, dates from about 3000 B.C. and there is a Babylonian physician's seal of approximately the same date in the Wellcome Historical Medical Museum, London. Epidemic fevers are mentioned in the Ebers papyrus, found in a tomb at Thebes by Professor Georg Ebers in 1862; the papyrus has been dated at 1500 B.C., but much of it was probably copied from an older work. In Exodus there is an account of the plague which smote Egypt about 1500 B.C., killing all the firstborn in the land, from the firstborn of Pharaoh on his throne to the firstborn of the captive in the dungeon and all the firstborn of cattle. This is one example of the effect of disease upon history, for the last terrible visitation upon the Egyptians persuaded Pharaoh to allow his Israelite slaves to depart; after forty years of wanderings and tribulations in the wilderness, they at last reached their promised land.

The war-pestilence sequence is well described in Samuel I. We are told that in 1141 B.C. the Israelites went out against the Philistines in battle, to be defeated with the loss of 4,000 men. The Israelites brought out their sacred Ark of the Covenant and re-engaged the Philistines, but suffered defeat and the loss of 30,000 men. The Philistines captured the Ark and bore it off to Ashdod, where plague at once broke out. The Ark was then removed—by public request—to Gath and thence to Ekron; both places were immediately smitten with plague. After seven months of suffering, the Philistines decided that their only hope was to return the Ark to Israel. It was delivered to the field of Joshua the Bethshemite, the return being greeted with sacrifices. But the curious Bethshemites looked into the Ark and were punished by a great pestilence which killed seventy men. It seems that the disease then spread throughout Israel, bringing death to about 50,000 people.

The plague of Athens in 430 B.C. provides a striking example of the effect of disease upon the course of history. At the beginning of the fifth century the Athenian empire was at the height of its power. This tiny Greek nation had defeated mighty Darius the Persian in the land battles of Marathon and Plataea and in the great naval engagement of Salamis. The enlightened reign of Pericles opened in 462 B.C.; under him the temples of Athens and Eleusis, destroyed by the Persians, were restored through the genius of the architect Ictinus and the artist Pheidias. But this golden age of Greece was all too brief. In 431 B.C. the Peloponnesian War started, an internecine struggle between the two main Hellenic powers of Athens and Sparta. Sparta was a military nation with a good army but no fleet; Athens a maritime power with a strong navy and a weak army. Since her land defences were almost invulnerable and ample supplies could be imported by sea, Athens could neither be brought to battle by land nor starved into submission. Fighting a defensive battle by land and an offensive war at sea, she should have been able to defeat Sparta without great difficulty. During the first year of the war the outcome seemed inevitable, for Athens was successful both on land and sea, but her defensive policy on land necessarily led to the Athenians being crowded and besieged within their city walls.

Disaster struck in 430 B.C. The pestilence is supposed to have started in Ethiopia; from there it travelled to Egypt and was carried across the Mediterranean by ship to the Piraeus and Athens. It raged for only a short time, but caused an enormous mortality. No estimate of the number of deaths can be made; perhaps at least a third and possibly as much as two-thirds of the population died. More disastrous still was the breakdown of morale, a not surprising phenomenon which we shall meet again in times of pandemic sickness. Thucydides, who left an account of this horrible time, wrote of the Athenians:

> ...fear of gods or law of men there was none to re-
> strain them. As for the first, they judged it to be just the
> same whether they worshipped them or not, as they saw
> all alike perishing; and as for the latter, no one expected
> to live to be brought to trial for his offences.

Thucydides added that even the most staid and respectable citizens devoted themselves to nothing but gluttony, drunkenness and licentiousness.

When it seemed that the plague had subsided, Pericles sent a powerful fleet to capture the Spartan-held stronghold of Potidaea. But, hardly had his navy set sail—or, to be accurate, rowed away—when plague broke out in the ships with such violence that the fleet was forced to return to Athens. A similar disaster occurred when Pericles himself led his fleet

7

to Epidauros, for 'the pestilence not only carried off his own men but all that had intercourse with them'. Pericles may have caught the infection at this time, for he is supposed to have died of plague in 429 B.C.

The nature of the visitation is unknown. The master physician Hippocrates, who lived at that time in Thessaly, left no description. Thucydides describes a very rapid onset, raging fever, extreme thirst, tongue and throat 'bloody', the skin of the body red and livid, finally breaking out into pustules and ulcers. The disease attacked all classes, rich and poor. Physicians were helpless and themselves succumbed in large numbers. The majority opinion holds that this was a highly malignant form of scarlet fever, probably the first appearance of the infection in the Mediterranean basin and therefore especially lethal. Other authorities have suggested bubonic plague, typhus, smallpox, measles, and anthrax of unusual virulence. There remains the possibility that the disease was one now unknown, but the balance of probability inclines to the first appearance of an epidemic infection which later became common and less fatal.

The plague of Athens undoubtedly contributed to the downfall of the Athenian empire. By killing so large a number, by demoralizing the capital and, above all, by destroying the fighting power of the navy, the plague prevented Athens striking a decisive blow at Sparta. The war dragged on for twenty-seven years and ended with the defeat of Athens in 404 B.C. She was deprived of her navy and of her foreign possessions and her landward fortifications were razed to the ground. Fortunately for posterity, the city and its culture were left intact.

Perhaps the most stupendous single event in history, in both the extent and longevity of its effect, is the downfall of the Roman empire. The causes of this fall have been argued by historians for many years past; but here we shall examine only such causes and effects connected with disease and its prevention.

Public health and sanitation were more advanced in the year A.D. 300 than they were to be again until the middle of the nineteenth century. The great drainage system, the Cloaca Maxima, was built in the sixth century B.C. to drain an area of marsh which later became the site of the Forum Romanum. The Cloaca gradually assumed the function of a modern sewer and its plan was copied elsewhere in Italy and the empire. The modern water closet was not devised until well over a thousand years after the fall of Rome, but the ruins of Pompeii and Herculaneum, destroyed by an eruption of Vesuvius in A.D. 79, have revealed an elaborate system of waterworks connected with flushing closets. Public lavatories, uncomfortably hard to find in the present-day city, were commonplace in Rome during the first century A.D. The best known of these, a palatial building fitted with marble urinals, was erected by the Emperor Vespasian in about A.D. 70; it is thought that there was a small charge for admission.

Cleanliness depends upon an adequate water supply. The first aqueduct brought pure water into Rome as early as 312 B.C. At the beginning of the Christian era there were six; a hundred years later no less than ten aqueducts supplied 250 million gallons of water daily. About half of this enormous supply was required for the public baths, but there remained fifty gallons per head for the 2 million inhabitants, the same amount that is used today by a citizen of New York or London. Some of these aqueducts have been repaired and are in use; in 1954 four aqueducts sufficed for the needs of modern Rome. The baths of Caracalla, dating from about A.D. 200, were capable of accepting 1,600 bathers at a time; those of Diocletian, built about eighty years later, had no less than 3,000 rooms. The bath, much like a modern sauna, accompanied Roman civilization wherever it penetrated, and certain places became famed for the curative power of their warm or mineral-impregnated waters. Some of these, such as Bath in England and Wiesbaden in Germany, retain a modest reputation as medicinal spas today.

The huge city-state of Rome had grown haphazardly, a town of crooked, narrow streets and squalid houses. Almost two-thirds of this was destroyed in A.D. 64 by the great fire in the reign of Nero. More fortunate than London after her fire,

Rome was rebuilt to a master plan, a city of straight, broad streets and wide squares. Cleaning of the public roads was supervised by the *aediles*, a body of officials who also controlled food supply. They introduced regulations to ensure the freshness and good quality of perishable foodstuffs, particularly meat, and they guarded against famine by storing vast quantities of corn, sometimes enough to supply the whole population for as long as ten years. Among other public health measures was the prohibition of burials within the city walls; the much more hygienic method of cremation became common and was not entirely replaced by burial until general acceptance of Christianity implanted the idea of physical resurrection.

In its cleanliness, sanitation and water supply, Rome was much more akin to twentieth-century London and New York than to mediaeval Paris or eighteenth-century Vienna. The Romans were the first urban-dwelling people on the grand scale; they must have dimly recognized, probably as the result of painful experience, that a large body of people cannot live closely together in health and with dignity if they lack a pure water supply, clean streets, and sewers. A seventeenth-century Londoner existed in conditions which would hardly have been tolerated by a first-century Roman, but they met on one common ground: neither knew the cause of disease. If the seemingly clean water that flowed along the Roman aqueduct happened to come from a contaminated source, then the Roman was as much at risk as the Londoner who drew his supply directly from the muddy Thames. This lack of essential knowledge rendered the magnificent health measures of Imperial Rome entirely useless during the long years of her plague-ridden decadence.

Imagine Rome as a bloated spider sitting in the centre of its web. That web, in the height of Roman expansion, stretched from the Sahara in the south to the borders of Scotland in the north, from the Caspian Sea and the Persian Gulf in the east to the western shores of Spain and Portugal. To north and west lay the oceans; to south and east, vast unknown continents in which dwelt less civilized peoples, Africans, Arabs, the savage tribes of Asia. Beyond, in the dim shadows, lay the older civilizations of India and China. The long land frontiers were manned by garrisons scattered at strategic points; from these frontier garrisons stretched back the filaments of the spider's web, the sea routes from Africa and Egypt, the straight, legionary-made roads, all of which led to Rome.

Herein lay the makings of disaster. A vast hinterland hiding unknown secrets, among them the micro-organisms of foreign disease; troops who attacked into that hinterland and were attacked by the inhabitants; free transit by ship or along roads specially built for speedy travel; at the centre a concentrated population living a highly civilized life yet lacking the most rudimentary means of combating infection. Given a conjunction of circumstances such as this, it is little wonder that the story of the last centuries of Roman power is a long tale of plague.

In the first century B.C. a very severe type of malaria appeared in the agricultural districts around Rome and remained a problem for the next 500 years. The ultimate effects of this invasion were probably more catastrophic than the attacks of Goths and Vandals. All the Campagna, the fertile land of market gardens which supplied the city with fresh vegetables, went out of cultivation; the small farmers who tilled it added to the overcrowding of Rome and, of course, brought the infection with them. It is primarily due to malaria, though there may have been other reasons as well, that the live-birth rate of the Italo-Romans fell steeply at a time when the birth rate throughout the conquered lands of the empire was rising. Further, the chronic weakness and ill-health caused by untreated malaria decreased life expectancy and enervated the nation. By the fourth century A.D., the mighty fighting power of the legions was no longer Italian; not only men but officers too were drawn from Germanic tribes. Possibly malaria, rather than decadent luxury imported from the East, accounted for the slackness of spirit which characterized the later years of Rome.

The second danger came from the remote East. Towards the end of the first century A.D. a warlike, merciless race, riding on stout ponies, emerged from the region of Mongolia over the steppes into south-east Europe. This exodus was probably dictated by disease or famine or by a combination of both in the lands north of China. Pressed by the invading Huns, the Germanic tribes of the central Euro-Asian land mass began a great westward movement. This relentless westward flow of Alans, Ostrogoths and Visigoths in the end submerged Rome and broke the close-knit empire into a rabble of warring states. During the years 451-4 the Huns themselves, under Attila, reached as far west as Orleans in Gaul and into northern Italy. They brought with them diseases unknown to Europe and may themselves have been turned back from Rome by the ravages of a disease unknown to them.

By her contacts with distant lands and peoples, Rome opened her gates to pestilence. The first of the great epidemics occurred about the year 79 A.D., shortly after the eruption of Vesuvius. This may have been fulminating malaria, possibly accompanied by an epidemic of anthrax which, being primarily a disease of animals, resulted in the large-scale destruction of livestock. The infection was confined to Italy, raging destructively in the cities, and causing some 10,000 deaths in the Campagna alone. For about a century there was much sickness, thought to have been chiefly malaria; then came the plague of Orosius in A.D. 125. This is an example of the famine-plague sequence, for the sickness was preceded by an invasion of locusts which destroyed large areas of crops. The pestilence that followed was particularly severe in Numidia, where 800,000 are reported to have died, and on the north coast of Africa where there was an estimated mortality of 200,000. The figures are probably exaggerated but suggest a high death roll. The plague passed from Africa to Italy, where so many died that whole villages and even towns were abandoned and fell to ruin.

Forty years later there followed the plague of Antoninus, sometimes known as the plague of the physician Galen. The story is better documented than that of previous outbreaks. Disease started among the troops of the co-emperor Lucius Verus on the eastern borders of the empire. It was confined to

12

the east for the two years 164-6 and caused great mortality among the legions under the command of Avidius Claudius, who had been sent to repress a revolt in Syria. The plague accompanied this army homewards, spreading throughout the countryside and reaching Rome in A.D. 166. It rapidly extended into all parts of the known world, causing so many deaths that loads of corpses were carried away from Rome and other cities in carts and wagons.

The plague of Antoninus or Galen, is notable because it caused the first crack in the Roman defence lines. Until A.D. 161 the empire continually expanded and maintained its frontiers. In that year a Germanic barbarian horde, the Marcomanni from Bohemia and the Quadi from Moravia, forced the north-eastern barrier of Italy. Owing to the fear and disorganization produced by the plague, full-scale retaliation could not be undertaken; not until A.D. 169 was the whole weight of Roman arms thrown against the Marcomanni. Possibly the failure of this invasion was as much due to the legions carrying plague with them as to their fighting prowess, for many Germans were found lying dead on the battlefield without sign of wounding. The pestilence raged until A.D. 180; one of the last victims was the noblest of Roman emperors, Marcus Aurelius. He died on the seventh day of his illness and is said to have refused to see his son at the last, fearing lest he, too, should succumb. After A.D. 180 there came a short respite followed by a return in 189. The spread of this second epidemic seems to have been less wide, but mortality in Rome was ghastly; as many as 2,000 sometimes died in a single day.

The name of the physician Galen is attached to the plague of A.D. 164-89 not only because he fled from it, but because he left a description of the disease. Initial symptoms were high fever, inflammation of the mouth and throat, parching thirst and diarrhoea. Galen described a skin eruption, appearing about the ninth day, sometimes dry and sometimes pustular. He implies that many patients died before the eruption appeared. There is here some resemblance to the Athenian plague, but the undoubted Eastern origin and the mention of pustules have led many historians to assert that this was the first instance of a smallpox epidemic. One theory holds that the westward movement of the Huns started because of virulent smallpox in Mongolia; the disease travelled with them, was communicated to the Germanic tribes upon whom the Huns were pressing and, in turn, infected the Romans who were in contact with the Germans. Against this theory must be set the fact that the later history of the Roman outbreak in no way resembles the later history of European smallpox in the sixteenth to nineteenth centuries. But, as we shall see in some of the following chapters, the first appearance of a disease often takes a form and a course which is quite different from that of the disease once established.

After A.D. 189, plague is not again mentioned until the year 250. Then appeared the great plague of Cyprian which indisputably changed the course of history. Its nature, however, is unknown. Cyprian, the Christian bishop of Carthage, described the symptoms as violent diarrhoea and vomiting, an ulcerated sore throat, burning fever, and putrefaction or gangrene of the hands and feet. Another account tells of a very rapid spread of disease all over the body and of unassuagable thirst. In neither account is there mention of any rash or skin eruption, unless the rapid spread 'all over the frame' be held to imply a visible manifestation of the disease. Like the Athenian plague, the place of origin is said to have been Ethiopia, from which it passed to Egypt and the Roman colonies in North Africa. North Africa was the granary of Rome; this fact, taken in conjunction with the mention of gangrenous hands and feet, tempts one to think of ergotism. Epidemic ergotism is caused by eating black bread made from rye which has been infected by the Claviceps fungus. But there is little evidence that rye, a crop of the north rather than of the south, was a staple bread corn of Rome, while the very wide spread and longevity of the plague of Cyprian are arguments against the theory. It is safer to leave the nature of the disease undefined.

The plague took the form of a true pandemic, spreading from Egypt in the south to Scotland in the north. It advanced with appalling speed, not only by contact with infected persons but by means of clothing or any other articles used by the sick. The first, devastating appearance was followed by a remission which ended with a renewed attack of equal virulence in the same district. There was a seasonal incidence, outbreaks starting in the autumn, lasting through winter and spring, and fading out with the coming of hot weather in summer. Mortality is said to have been higher than in any other pestilence, the deaths of infected persons outnumbering those who survived attack. The plague of Cyprian lasted for no less than sixteen years, during which time something in the nature of a general panic developed. Thousands fled the countryside to overcrowd cities and so cause fresh outbreaks; wide areas of farmland throughout Italy reverted to waste; some thought that the human race could not possibly survive. Despite warfare in Mesopotamia, on the eastern frontiers and even in Gaul, the empire managed to survive this catastrophe; but by A.D. 275 the legions had fallen back from Transylvania and the Black Forest to the Danube and the Rhine, and so dangerous did the position seem to have become that Aurelian decided to fortify the city of Rome itself.

Throughout the next three centuries, while Rome slowly collapsed under the pressure of Goth and Vandal, there were recurrent outbreaks of a similar plague. Gradually the evidence becomes less exact, degenerating into a generalized story of war, pestilence and famine, as the darkness descended over Rome and her mighty empire disintegrated. The Germanic peoples crowded into Italy, Gaul, across the Pyrenees into Spain, even into North Africa, where plague so weakened the Vandals in A.D. 480 that they were unable to resist a later invasion by Moors. There are rumours of a great mortality in Rome (467) and around Vienna in 455. Of special interest, because it may have affected the history of the Anglo-Saxons, is a visitation in Britain, apparently part of a general pandemic in 444. According to Bede, mortality was so great in Britain that barely enough healthy men survived to bury the dead, while the plague depleted the forces of the Romano-British chieftain Vortigern to such an extent that he was unable to cope with the incursions of the savage Picts and Scots. Legend relates that, after taking counsel with his chieftains, Vortigern decided to seek help from the Saxons, who in 449 arrived in Britain as mercenaries under their leaders Hengist and Horsa. It may indeed have been plague which so weakened the British that Saxon infiltration was successful.

Meanwhile a new Roman empire had arisen in the East. Asia Minor had been annexed to Rome in the first century B.C. Four hundred years later Constantine the Great founded his eastern capital at Byzantium. One hundred and fifty years later the Western empire of Rome was in process of complete disintegration, but the Eastern empire of Byzantium survived as a ruling power until the Frankish conquest of 1204. Byzantium maintained the fabric of Roman government; more, Byzantium cherished the dream of resurrecting Rome and reuniting the Western with the Eastern empire. This dream was almost translated into reality by the great Emperor Justinian. After securing peace on his eastern and northern borders, Justinian launched an attack on the west in A.D. 532. He recaptured Carthage and much of the north coast of Africa, retook Sicily, and crossed to Italy. Naples fell to his general Belisarius; undefended Rome, Ravenna, all central and southern Italy were captured by the imperial armies. In A.D. 540 it seemed that Germanic resistance had been broken; Justinian, having also reconquered part of Spain, began to form bold plans to carry his conquests into Gaul and even into Britain.

His victories brought no lasting gain. The Moors drove the Byzantines from most of the African seaboard; in 541 a brilliant young Goth leader, Totila, won back the greater part of Italy. Totila was willing to come to terms with Justinian, but the emperor had determined upon conquest. There followed eleven years of bitter warfare in which Rome underwent siege five times. At the end of the war she had become a city of a few thousand impoverished inhabitants set in a desert of malarial wastes. During one of their sieges, the Goths cut the aqueducts in an endeavour to force surrender. Mediaeval squalor and uncleanliness derive in part from this act because

16

Rome, with her magnificent buildings and historical prestige, never wholly lost her influence upon the Western world. If she had still had a functioning and plentiful supply of clean water other European cities might have made a similar provision.

The reign of Justinian should have been a time of imperial splendour. He girdled his domains with a chain of castles and forts; he erected many magnificent buildings, including the cathedral of St Sophia. His code of laws, which embodied those of ancient Rome, was to form the basis of European justice for centuries to come. He recruited excellent armies, especially skilled pikemen and bowmen, which were commanded by successful generals such as Belisarius and Narses. Yet, during his reign, the Huns very nearly succeeded in taking his capital, the Slavs captured Adrianople and the Persians sacked Antioch. His government, which had begun in a blaze of glory, steadily declined. When Justinian died in A.D. 565 at the age of eighty-three, he left his empire considerably poorer and weaker than when he had mounted the throne in 527. For in 540, the year of his greatest success, an enemy more fearful than Goth or Vandal lay in wait for him.

The plague of Justinian may have been the most terrible that has ever harrowed the world. We know something of it from the account written by Procopius, the secretary or archivist of Justinian's reign. It started in A.D. 540 at Pelusium in Lower Egypt, spreading throughout Egypt to Alexandria and to Palestine. Palestine seems to have been the focus of spread to the rest of the known world. It reached Byzantium in the spring of 542. The mortality was not at first great but rapidly rose until some 10,000 died each day. So many were the deaths that graves could not be dug sufficiently quickly. Roofs were taken off the towers of forts, the towers filled with corpses and the roofs replaced. Ships were loaded with the dead, rowed out to sea and abandoned.

This sickness was undoubtedly bubonic plague. Victims were seized with sudden fever; on the first or second day buboes, swollen glands, appeared in the groin or armpit. Many patients became deeply comatose, others developed a

17

violent delirium in which they saw phantoms or heard voices prophesying death; sometimes the buboes broke down into gangrenous sores and the sufferer died in terrible pain. Death usually occurred on the fifth day, but could be very quick or delayed for a week or two. Physicians were unable to tell which cases were light and which severe; as there was no known remedy, they were quite useless. Procopius makes two points. First, he states that the plague always began on the coast and spread inland. Second, he says that it was not contagious for, contrary to expectation, doctors or attendants who nursed the sick and laid out the dead, did not fall victims more readily than others.

The plague returned again and again, lasting until about the year 590. It spared no town or village, but ravaged even the most remote settlements; if a region seemed to have escaped, the plague would surely appear in due time. As in the plague of Cyprian, there was a seasonal occurrence and an outbreak might fade for a few years only to recur in the same place with equal ferocity. All ages were at risk but more men died than women. Many cities and villages were wiped out or abandoned, agriculture largely ceased, panic threw the whole empire into confusion. Gibbon states that entire countries never regained their previous density of population. Procopius makes the observation, common to so many plague chronicles, that the depravity and licentiousness after the pestilence suggested that only the most wicked had been spared.

The extent to which plague contributed to the downfall of Rome and to the wreck of Justinian's ambitions must be an open question. Incurable infectious disease is no respecter of persons; it ravages impartially the highly civilized and the less civilized. But the city dweller is at greater risk than the countryman and, in a mortal epidemic, a close-knit organization will disintegrate more easily than a loose association. Of supreme importance is the fact that failure of morale is more likely to occur among those who have lived softly than among men who have known hardship all their lives. Thus, although pestilence must have affected the fighting power of the savage

18

tribes, its impact upon Roman and Byzantine life was immeasurably greater. When we consider the frightful sequence of pestilences that smote the empire during the time of its decadence we need hardly search for a more potent cause of disaster.

Besides undermining the Roman state, the plague visitations of the first three centuries A.D. produced two far-reaching and long-lasting effects which are less widely recognized. First, Christianity would hardly have succeeded in establishing itself as a world force, and would certainly not have taken the form that it has, if the Roman empire had not been ravaged by incurable disease during the years which followed the life of Christ. Second, the thousand-year history of medicine from the fourth until the fourteenth century would have been very different had not medicine fallen under the domination of the Christian church. To understand what happened we must go back to the beginnings of European civilization, when priest and doctor were one and the same.

In the early, misty days of Greek legend, the god Apollo was born of the goddess Leto on the island of Delos. Apollo was carried to Delphi, where he killed a great snake, a very ancient symbol of disease. By this act, Apollo became the god of health, but he was also the bringer of pestilence, which he visited on mortals by means of the arrows which he loosed. He must therefore be not only worshipped but also placated. Apollo passed the secrets of the healing art to Chiron, a centaur, who in turn instructed Jason, Achilles and Asklepios or Aesculapius. The latter (who may actually have lived, at about 1250 B.C.) was so successful as a physician, even restoring the dead to life, that the god Zeus became alarmed at the diminishing supply of souls to the underworld and slew him with a thunderbolt. Aesculapius was honoured as a god and worshipped in hundreds of temples throughout Hellas.

As the cult of Aesculapius grew, it developed into the ritual of incubation or temple-sleep. The patient made sacrifice to the healing god and purified himself by bathing (lustration). Then he lay down to sleep in a long open corridor; here Aesculapius might appear to the sufferer in a dream and give advice, or his sacred serpents might effect a cure by licking the patient's sores or his eyes. In later years the magical temple-sleep was reinforced by physical therapy: exercise, diet, massage and bathing. Many patients stayed in the temples for weeks or even months; the temple developed into something closely akin to the nineteenth-century 'hydropathic' and the treatment was no doubt equally successful.

The Greeks evolved the 'scientific approach'. Pythagoras (580-498 B.C.) is the father of mathematics, but he also founded a system of medicine. Among his pupils were two physicians, Alcmaeon and Empedocles, who enunciated the doctrine of the four elements, earth, water, fire and air, and produced theories of respiration, sight, hearing and brain function. Their teaching was elaborated by Hippocrates (460-355 B.C.), one of the great figures of the golden age of Pericles. Hippocrates believed that the human body was made up of four humours, blood, phlegm, yellow and black bile, and could be predominantly hot, cold, moist or dry. He denied that disease was a punishment sent by the gods, and is regarded by many as the founder of the medical art.

By 355 B.C., medicine had ceased to be pure thaumaturgy and had acquired a rational basis, but how far this 'scientific approach' affected the actual practice must remain problematical. Hippocrates cannot have been only a theorist; he described recognizable diseases and the results of treatment. But the cult of Aesculapius certainly survived Hippocrates and it is noticeable that the great physician claimed—or the claim was made on his behalf—that he was a direct descendant of Aesculapius. There is no certainty that Hippocrates founded a school; the first known semblance of a medical school is that of Alexandria, founded twenty years after his death. It is unlikely that his teachings spread widely or that his influence was great during his lifetime.

This point is of importance in the history of Roman medicine. According to Pliny the Elder, the Romans got on very well without doctors for 600 years. There was medicine of a kind: the head of the family treated his descendants with folk remedies and sacrificial rites were accorded to the appropriate god. Both Apollo and Aesculapius had their votaries, for Rome borrowed from all countries, but there were many native demigods, a number of whom were directly concerned with disease: Salus and Mars ruled health in general, Carmenta looked after childbirth, Febris was the goddess of fever, Mephitis of disease-producing airs, Carna goddess of the stomach. It has been said that the Romans possessed an appropriate god for every function of life, for every part of the body, for every natural phenomenon, and that each god must be placated by his or her own particular and exact ritual. If the favour sought was not received, the wrong god had been called upon or the incorrect rite performed.

The practice of medicine was beneath the dignity of a Roman citizen. The first physicians were slaves of Greek extraction. About 220 B.C., over a hundred years after the death of Hippocrates, the first of these Greek physicians, a man named Archagethes, appeared in Rome. He was followed by many more, but none lived up to the standards of Hippocrates; they seem to have been more interested in money than their patients' welfare. The physicians were granted the freedom of Rome by no less a man than Julius Caesar and their standing was bettered under Augustus but, so far as is known, medical practice always remained in the hands of foreigners. When malaria and plague visited the Roman empire, the suffering population could call upon only their ancient gods or the Greek physicians. Neither was outstandingly successful, so it is not surprising that the Romans sought help elsewhere.

Because of her contacts with foreign nations and because of her almost unlimited pantheism, Rome sheltered and tolerated a great variety of religions. Not only had she her own domestic gods, but she drew on the deities of Greece and of the East. Among the conquered peoples whose religions became influential were the Jews. Small Jewish communities were scattered throughout the length of the Mediterranean seaboard and the number of these communities increased after the Dispersion following the war of A.D. 66.

These Jewish communities were renowned for their moral

way of life, their upright dealing, their charities, their care of the sick and poor. Many Gentiles found themselves attracted to the Jewish way of living. But their religious practices proved a barrier. In the words of Henry Chadwick, the Jews

> ... would not be associated either directly or indirectly with any pagan cult (which seemed antisocial), they refused to eat not only meat that had been offered in sacrifice to the gods but also all pork (which seemed ridiculous, and they circumcised their male infants (which seemed repulsive).

The more liberal Jewish communities did not insist that the Gentile follow these strange rites, but permitted him to enter an outer circle of 'God-fearers' and to attach himself to the synagogue. The earliest Christian missionaries, among them the apostle Paul, found their first converts in the 'God-fearers' and it was in these para-Jewish congregations that the Christians of the Roman empire first established themselves. This is why, for purposes of toleration or persecution, Jew and Christian were one and the same in the eyes of official Rome.

During the first century after the birth of Christ, His immediate followers, the apostles, were still living. Teaching was oral and the doctrines of Christianity as yet unformed. During the second century, the basic pattern of Christian doctrine began to be summarized in creeds and the text of the New Testament. The three synoptic gospels of Matthew, Mark and Luke mention a number of 'miracles' performed by Christ. Twenty of these miracles are described by Luke; two more, the walking on the waters and the strange cursing of the barren fig-tree, are not in Luke. If we analyse Luke's miracles, we find that there are only three—the quietening of the storm, the miraculous draught of fishes, and the feeding of the multitude—which are not of a medical nature. In four cases unclean spirits are cast out, in two the dead are restored to life, and in eleven sickness or disability is cured. In addition Luke positively states: 'He called the twelve together and gave them power and authority over all devils, and to cure diseases.' This authority was later extended to the seventy disciples. Thus the miraculous and divine healing power was transferred to the followers of Christ.

The second century A.D. was a time of mortal sickness, with the plague of Orosius in 125 and that of Antoninus which lasted from 164 until 180. To the terror-stricken victims of these visitations, Christianity offered new hope that was not to be found in any other creed. There was the promise of physical resurrection after death, coupled with the surety of ultimate bliss for the sinner who truly repented. Above all, for the living, the miracles of Christ and the miraculous power entrusted by him to his followers were an earnest of divine intervention which might cure mortal sickness or defeat death itself. Thus, the growth of the Christian Church was stimulated by its specific medical mission in a succession of plagues. By the middle years of the third century, the small scattered Christian communities had coalesced into an established Church, and this process was greatly accelerated by the plague of Cyprian in 250. Conversions were more numerous at all times of famine, earthquake or pestilence; at the height of the plague of Cyprian he and his fellow priests in North Africa were baptizing as many as two or three hundred persons a day.

So was formed the cult of Christ the Healer. The third-century persecutions of Decius and Diocletian failed to stamp out Christianity and it received imperial sanction from Constantine the Great in 313; at the end of the fourth century Christianity was adopted as the official religion of the empire after the enactment of laws against paganism by Theodosius. About this time, or perhaps a little before, the practice of medicine passed into the hands of the Church; under the Byzantine emperors, priest and doctor once more became the same. The Christian followed the Jew in his care of the sick. It is not quite true to say that the Christians were the first to found hospitals, for camp infirmaries existed under the Roman republic and the great hospital of Bartholomew on the Tiber dates from 293 B.C. But sick-nursing became a Christian duty and, as communities dedicated to service were founded, the infirmary formed an essential part of commu-

nity life. Early hospitals and early churches were designed
upon the same plan: a central altar with two or four long
naves or wards leading from it, and a number of side wards
or chapels, each placed under the patronage of a saint. In
these hospitals, treatment was in the hands of priests, assisted
by lay brethren and sisters, who combated disease almost
wholly by appeal to supernatural agency.

The approach of the Byzantine and mediaeval 'doctor' was
essentially the same as that of the present-day Christian
Scientist. Disease was a punishment, resulting from sin, a
lapse from the purity of Christian life. The cure, if God decided to effect a cure, could only be by miraculous intervention.
But the cure did not necessarily come from God alone. Just
as the demigods of pagan Rome had intervened to affect the
course of disease, so the demigods or saints of the Christian
church could be invoked to perform a miracle. Some of these
demigods or saints were physicians credited with special
powers, like the martyrs Cosmas and Damien, twin brothers
who practised medicine without charging fees and were put
to death during one of the early persecutions. They may have
been a christianized version of the pagan Dioscuri, twin sons
of Zeus, or they may have been living persons. Cosmas and
Damien suffered martyrdom by being tied to stakes and
stoned to death; miraculously restored, their lives were ended
by decapitation. Their story embodies the themes of self-
sacrifice, patient suffering, resurrection and then final death
common to many of the Christian patrons of disease.

Other medical saints are Roman demigods who, under
altered names, were assigned patronage of various diseases
and bodily parts or functions. Febris, the goddess of fever,
barely changed her name to become St Febronia. St Blaise, a
bishop and martyr about whom nothing factual is known,
looked after the throat; St Apollonia became the patron of
toothache because her own teeth were knocked out by an
anti-Christian mob at Alexandria in A.D. 249; St Erasmus of
Elmo took over the charge of the abdomen from the demi-
goddess Carna because he suffered martyrdom in 303 by
having his intestines drawn out with a windlass. St Lawrence

became patron of the back on the rather slender grounds that, when roasted to death on a gridiron in 258, he had asked to be turned over as his back was now quite done. St Lucy, martyred in 304, guarded the eyes; she later became confused with St Triduana of Scotland who, when her eyes were admired by a pagan lover, plucked them out and presented them to him impaled on a skewer.

Among saints who were invoked against special diseases are St Dympna, the entirely mythical patroness of insanity; a thirteenth-century asylum dedicated to her still exists at Gheel near Antwerp. Another quite mythical person, St Avertin, became patron of epilepsy. People who suffered from haemorrhoids, or piles, turned to the sixth-century Irish St Fiacre, who was also the patron saint of gardeners and later gave his name to the Paris cab. Better known is St Vitus, said to have been a youth martyred under Diocletian, who gave his name to St Vitus's Dance, a term commonly applied nowadays to chorea. St Anthony, a hermit born near Memphis in 251 and dying when 104 years of age, is associated with St Anthony's Fire, which may have been erysipelas, bubonic plague, typhus or ergotism.

Of special interest is the legend of St Sebastian, the patron of epidemic pestilence. His entirely mythical history illustrates the transference of miraculous power from the Roman or Greek demigod to the Christian saint. His biography relates that Sebastian was born of noble parents at Narbonne in the third century. At an early age he commanded a company of the Praetorian Guard and was constantly about the person of the Emperor Diocletian. Although remaining loyal to his emperor, Sebastian secretly became a Christian and converted others, including two noble youths, Marcus and Marcellinus. These two were accused, confessed under torture, and were led out to die. Their parents implored them to recant; Sebastian so exhorted them that not only did they refuse, but their guards and their judges were converted. A few months later, in 288, all these were tried and condemned. Diocletian himself urged recantation on Sebastian and, when he refused, ordered him to be tied to a stake and shot to death with arrows. This order was carried out and Sebastian was left for dead. At midnight Irene, the widowed mother of either Marcus or Marcellinus, found him still alive and nursed him back to health. His friends then pleaded with Sebastian to leave Rome; he refused, stationed himself at the palace gate, and pleaded with Diocletian to spare his fellow Christians. Diocletian thereupon ordered Sebastian to be taken to the circus and flogged to death. His body was thrown into the Cloaca Maxima, but, following a vision vouchsafed to the Christian Lucinda, was recovered and buried in the catacombs, above which the church of St Sebastiano now stands.

The cult of St Sebastian as patron of epidemic sickness started about the year 680. The earliest representations of Sebastian depict him as an elderly, bearded man, fully clothed; in one such painting he is turning the arrows aside with a fold of his cloak. Later pictures show him as a youth of great physical beauty, naked except for a loincloth. The inference is that Sebastian had become identified with Apollo. There is also the symbolism of the arrow: the arrows of Apollo were the conveyors of disease and Sebastian miraculously survived them; thus, as one who had survived the arrows of disease, St Sebastian was empowered to protect and restore others who had been so attacked.

Christian treatment of disease borrowed largely from Graeco-Roman practice. The sacrificial offering to the demigod became the votive offering to the saint. The temple-sleep or incubation of the Asclepeiad remained unchanged, but the devotee looked for the appearance of healing saints, especially Cosmas and Damien, in his dreams. Lustration, the ritual washing of the Aesculapeian cult, formed an essential part of Christian treatment but was rapidly degraded from a beneficial cleansing of the body into a ceremonial sprinkling with holy water, a custom still observed in the Roman Catholic and Orthodox churches. Binding and loosing, a practice particularly associated with the goddess Carna (who started as warden of the lock and key, then of the lying-in room, and so of the abdomen) in Roman times became manual hypnosis and was transformed by the Christian priest into the laying

26

on of hands, still practised by those who call themselves 'spiritual healers'.

So the cult of Christ the Healer was an essential aspect of both the work and the faith of the early Church. It is no blasphemy to acknowledge and to honour Jesus Christ as one of the greatest and most successful founders of a new system of medicine. But his followers were psychiatrists and faith-healers rather than physicians. The theocratic 'physician' of Christian Byzantium and the later monastic infirmarian depended primarily upon supernatural intervention and only secondarily upon mundane treatment. Much of that treatment itself was frank magic: the swallowing of written paternosters or fragments of alleged saintly bone, prayer, penitence, fasting and votive offering. But there existed a solid foundation of psychological medicine and there was also a rational basis of medical theory, of anatomy, and of physical treatment.

If Christ was the founder of the Christian school of medicine, Galen was its acknowledged authority and unchallenged teacher. This is strange, for Galen was not a Christian, although he seems to have defended Christianity and to have preferred a theoretical monotheism to the Roman welter of demigods. Born about the year A.D. 131 at Pergamos in Asia Minor, Galen was appointed surgeon to the gladiators there and later removed to Rome. Here he practised and taught medicine, conducted a number of scientific experiments, and acquired a great reputation. It is said that he fled the city during the plague of 166-180 which bears his name, but was recalled by Marcus Aurelius to Rome, where he died in 200. A forceful, dogmatic teacher, Galen is thought to have written some 500 treatises on medical and scientific subjects, only a small fraction of which have survived. He made many advances in anatomy, physiology, and medicine but he fouled the earlier and simpler methods of treatment with a vast collection of noisome and useless remedies. Hence came the vile mixtures, often containing as many as fifty or sixty ingredients, by which mediaeval practitioners are somewhat unjustly remembered.

For nearly twelve hundred years and throughout the whole of the Dark Ages, the lamp of Greek medicine flickered on in scattered monasteries and in those small islands of culture which successfully withstood the general decline that followed the end of Imperial Rome. On the other side of the Mediterranean, in Alexandria, the school of the so-called Arabian physicians, many of whom were Jews and Christians, added something to medical advance. They, too, had learned from the followers of Christ, for their knowledge derived from the congregation of Nestorius, the Christian Patriarch of Jerusalem who had been banished for heresy in 431. The Arabs revered Galen but, more liberal than the Christians, they questioned, tested, and recast his theories. In the end, these two schools merged into one, but this was not to happen fully until the change in habits of thought which ushered in the Renaissance at the beginning of the fifteenth century. By that time the Church's domination of medicine had become repressive and the influence of Galen had waxed so great that to question his authority was no less than heresy.

2

The Black Death

The Black Death was a type of bubonic plague. The plague of Justinian was undoubtedly bubonic plague and a good case can be put forward for the plague of the Philistines being the same disease. According to Samuel I, verses 4-5, the Philistines were advised to placate the Israelite God with talismanic offerings:

> What shall be the trespass offering which we shall return to him? They answered Five golden emerods and five golden mice ... images of your emerods and images of your mice that mar the land.

The Authorized Version of the Old Testament states that

the 'emerods' which smote the Philistines 'in their secret parts' is an archaic term for 'piles' but the Revised Version has the translation 'tumours'; 'mice' may be a mistranslation of 'rats'. It has been suggested that the disease was dysentery rather than bubonic plague, but the hazards of mistranslation are so great that it is impossible to state a definite opinion.

The term 'bubonic' refers to the characteristic bubo or enlarged lymphatic gland. Bubonic plague is primarily a disease of rodents. The most common carrier is the rat. Bubonic plague is passed from rat to rat by the fleas which infest them. The flea bites an infected rat and ingurgitates plague bacilli. These bacilli can remain in the flea's intestinal canal for as long as three weeks and are regurgitated when the flea bites a man. In true bubonic plague, man will become infected only if fleas migrate from rodents to humans or from human to human. Bubonic plague is not carried by the patient's breath or by direct contact.

The common source of infection is the black rat (*Rattus rattus*) sometimes known as the Old English Rat. This animal is companionable with man. It is a rather handsome beast, with silky black fur, and, unlike the brown rat, tends to live in houses or ships rather than in farmyards or sewers. This companionship with man makes migration of fleas from rats to humans easy and so permits the spread of bubonic plague. The disease, whether of rat or man, has a very high mortality rate; 90 per cent of infected cases has been recorded in some epidemics. In man, the plague is typically seen as buboes, enlarged glands usually occurring in the groin (the 'secret parts' of the Bible story) but also in the armpit or neck. The causative organism, *Pasteurella pestis*, rapidly multiplies in the bloodstream, causing a high temperature and death from septicaemia (blood poisoning).

So far the story suggests a dangerous disease, not very common, occurring in isolated cases or in small sporadic epidemics. This is the kind of picture seen in countries where bubonic plague is endemic today, and is also true of Europe from about A.D. 600 until 1700. But there are two other forms of the disease: septicaemic, in which a rapidly fatal septi-caemia occurs before buboes have a chance to develop; and pneumonic, in which the signs and symptoms are those of an exceptionally virulent pneumonia. All three types can occur separately or together, but it is the last that primarily concerns us here, for pneumonic plague can spread directly from man to man without transmission by rat or flea. The breath and the sputum of the victim of pneumonic plague are quite literally crowded with bacilli; as he speaks, coughs, sneezes he will scatter these bacilli far and wide and any bystander will be in danger of inhaling them into his own lungs and so developing the pneumonic type of bubonic plague himself.

In this form plague can spread widely and rapidly. One sporadic case of the pneumonic type may cause a pandemic. But the reason why this occurrence is so rare remains a mystery. In the 1,100 years between 540 and 1666 there have been only three great pandemics, the plague of Justinian of 540-90, the Black Death of 1346-61, and that which raged in Europe during the years 1665-6 and produced the so-called Great Plague of London. In the plague of Justinian and the plague of 1665, the pandemic started as a rat-flea-man infection. The spread was inland from the coast and those who attended the sick were at no greater risk than those who did not; in Byzantium the death rate was small at the beginning but rapidly rose to an appalling figure. The same pattern is seen in 1665. Pepys noted 'much against my will' that two or three houses in Drury Lane were marked with a red cross on 7 June, 1665; from 7 June until 1 July, the weekly return of plague deaths was 100, 300, 450, but thereafter the rise was increasingly steep, reaching 2,000 by the end of July, 6,500 at the end of August, and over 7,000 at the peak in the third week of September. The estimated population of London in 1665 was 460,000 and bubonic plague was only rarely entirely absent from the city. A rise of the death rate to 200 to 300 a week can be attributed to a great increase in the number of infected rats, but a mortality of thousands argues a direct man-to-man infection. Thus at some point in the plague of Justinian and the plague of 1665 the mode of trans-

31

mission must have changed from the rat-flea-man cycle of bubonic plague to the predominantly pneumonic type. The same must be true of the Black Death.

Reaching southward into Africa, eastward to China, and northward to Russia and the Scandinavian countries, the Black Death was a world-wide pandemic. Indeed, it is just possible that the devastation wrought in Scandinavia may ultimately have had a greater effect upon world history than did the English catastrophe. Ships carried infection to the Greenland settlements founded by Erik the Red in A.D. 936. These colonies were so weakened by the plague and by failure of supplies from enfeebled Norway that they could not withstand Eskimo attacks. The last Viking settlers disappeared in the fifteenth century and Greenland became unknown country until rediscovered by John Davis in 1585. It is thought that the Viking settlements maintained sporadic contact with 'Vinland', which was part of the coast of Canada or Newfoundland, so the Black Death may have entirely altered the history of North America.

Its impact upon the future of England was greater than upon any other European country. The reason is that the English social system was already showing signs of strain and the Black Death accelerated its collapse. In Europe the system was more rigid and survived for many years. At the beginning of the fourteenth century England was governed by the feudal system, of which it has been said that everything ultimately belonged to someone else. The great lord held his lands from the king; the knight held his manor from the lord; the smaller landowner from the knight, and the villein from the village landowner. Rental was paid by service. Thus the baron owed so many knights to the crown, the knight so many men-at-arms to his lord, while the peasant was forced to work so many days upon his lord's land before he might till his own. This, of course, is an over-simplification; the system was far more complex and less complete in practice. One complication was the existence of money; so long as money was in very short supply and confined to the ruling class, the basic principle could be fairly widely applied.

But, when coin entered into more general circulation, there developed a tendency to commute service for cash; the lord stayed at home instead of leading his knights; the knight found it more profitable to leave his tenant farmers to till the land and to pay a small force of professional soldiers; even the peasant sometimes managed to commute his service for rent or to demand a wage for additional labour. A growing population brought into being a quite large class of landless workers; these had to be paid in coin for their toil.

Thus an increased flow of money weakened feudalism. The great agricultural boom of the thirteenth century led to an excess of crops over and above the level necessary for national subsistence. The upper classes and especially the Church, the largest landowner in the country, devoted themselves with energy and intelligence to the business of farming. Trade and industry had developed since the days of the Norman, but agriculture remained the predominant and most gainful occupation of England.

By the end of the thirteenth century more land in England had been brought under plough than ever before and possibly than ever since. England had become a grain-exporting country, sending a steady supply of bread corns—wheat from the south, barley and oats from the north—to the Continent in the small ships of her merchant fleet. This corn had to be collected in centres, the market towns and manorial barns, before being carried by wagon to the ports. The heavy wagons demanded well-maintained roads; for this reason the road system of England was in better condition and travel was easier in 1300 than at any time until the end of the eighteenth century. The agricultural boom allowed a high standard of living and this, in turn, affected the live-birth rate and expectation of life. Population steadily increased from less than 2 million at the time of the Norman Conquest to at least $3\frac{1}{2}$ million and perhaps more nearly 5 million in 1300.

Corn exports allowed not only luxury imports but an increase in coin. Because of a flourishing agriculture and because of the wider distribution of money, there was considerable buying and selling of land by free peasants and exchange or leasing by the unfree as early as the thirteenth century. But the fact that a peasant possessed money did not necessarily mean that he could become a free man. His chances of freedom depended upon local conditions. Generally speaking, it was easier in the north, which was more remote from the Continental market and where there was less arable land requiring a large labour force.

By the end of the thirteenth century the basically simple structure of the feudal state had been complicated by a number of variants. The greatest weakness and the greatest danger to stability lay in the anomaly that the poorer peasants of the less highly cultivated areas had the better chance of freedom, while the more wealthy peasants of the predominantly arable counties found their bondage increased.

These peasants constituted the large majority of the English people and were the class most profoundly affected by the Black Death. The richer classes lived their lives apart, travelling quite widely, enjoying the benefits of imported goods, dwelling in stone houses which often boasted chimneys and glazed windows. Many of their houses are scattered throughout the English countryside of today, some of them picturesque ruins, a few still inhabited. The peasant's house has almost entirely disappeared. Most lived in a round, tent-like cot, built of poles filled in with clay and brushwood, thatched with heather, straw or reed, with no chimney and no windows. The peasant's diet was probably fairly good but there were great variations, both regional and seasonal, and times of dearth following bad seasons must have been not infrequent. The staple foods were grain products, honey, bacon, peas and beans. Fresh vegetables, with the possible exception of leeks and the cabbage-like collards, could only be obtained in summer. Lack of winter feed prevented the keeping of more than a few head of cattle from year to year, so dairy products, with the exception of a little cheese, were also summer foodstuffs. Lack of fresh meat, absence of milk and butter during the winter months, a deficiency of fresh vegetables coupled with the curious fact that fruit was generally regarded as unwholesome, rendered the peasant liable

34

to the vitamin-deficiency diseases, particularly scurvy. He ate well during the summer and autumn, but the long winter and spring months were a time of undernourishment, aggravated by the cold and damp of his working conditions and of his housing.

Failure of a harvest resulted in widespread starvation. The village community might be able to survive by snaring a few birds, poaching wild rabbits, and scratching the scanty resources of woodland and field: nuts, grasses, docks and nettles. But only the able-bodied could hope to live through a prolonged period of extreme scarcity until the new harvest brought fresh supplies. The very young and the elderly died of frank malnutrition or of intercurrent disease against which their enfeebled bodies could offer little resistance. The ills of damp and cold, particularly lung infections, must have carried off many older people and young children at these times; this was symptomatic of a general diminution of resistance which rendered the whole community more liable to attack by infectious disease. It seems that famine-sickness occurred on a major scale only once (1257-9) during the agricultural prosperity of the thirteenth century, but with the opening of the fourteenth century and the end of the boom years there came a recession which exerted a profound effect upon England's health and economy.

Extensive dairy farming and meat production were impossible because of the difficulty of keeping beasts through the winter, so the great landlords turned to sheep. A fair amount of wool was already being produced for home use in the twelfth century, but now the change from arable to sheep started to accelerate. As a result, the standard of living of the peasantry began to fall and the birth rate declined. The economic standard of the peasant was further weakened by the war against the Scots in 1296 and by the Hundred Years War against the French which began in 1327. The Continental campaigns of Edward II, especially, could not be sustained by feudal levy and demanded paid or 'indentured' troops, whose cost ultimately fell upon the man who tilled the soil.

Thus in the year 1346 the outwardly stable structure of the

feudal system had developed a number of cracks, the economy of the realm was shaky, and the subsistence level of the peasantry lay at the mercy of a bad harvest. A network of quite good roads linked inland towns and villages to the Channel and North Sea ports; a stream of fighting men passed backwards and forwards across a short sea route to the battlefields of France. Given the sequence of a bad harvest, a famine-stricken populace, and a pestilence on the continent of Europe, spread of disease throughout England was inevitable. That sequence occurred in the years 1347 and 1348.

Men look back on world-shaking events to remember that they were preceded by signs and wonders in the heavens. There are reports of earthquakes, eruptions, tidal waves, in the years immediately preceding the Black Death but these, if they occurred at all, are coincidental. The one reported antecedent which had some effect upon the course of the pestilence is a quite appalling weather pattern which seems to have been general throughout Europe during the years 1346-8. The series of three abnormally wet and cold summers, culminating in that of 1348, when it is related that rain fell unceasingly from midsummer until Christmas, imply a period of prolonged dearth with consequent malnutrition, illness and reduced resistance to infectious disease.

The Black Death probably first broke out in the small fortified trading-post of Caffa (now Theodosia) on the Crimean shore of the Black Sea. In 1344 a company of Italian merchants, engaged in the overland trade between Europe and China, had taken refuge here from attack by a Tartar horde. The Tartars settled down to besiege the place, but the Italians successfully repelled them for over two years. This besieging army was probably reinforced from time to time by new bands from southern Russia and the East. According to one account, plague broke out in Caffa itself during the winter of 1346-7; a second story relates that it was introduced into the fort by the besiegers by means of corpses thrown over the walls. Both sides suffered many deaths and the siege was raised. The Tartar horde dispersed, carrying the plague with them to the Caspian Sea; thence it spread northward to

Russia and eastward to India and China, where it first arrived in 1352. Such of the Italian traders as still survived escaped from Caffa by ship for Genoa. The chronicler Gabriel De Mussis stated that no case of plague occurred on the voyage but that it appeared at Genoa in a deadly form a day or two after the ship docked. His statement suggests that the disease was still in its rat-flea-man cycle.

From its European source in Genoa the plague quickly swept in a great west and north half-circle through Italy, France, Germany and the Scandinavian countries to join up with the slower northern invasion, reaching Moscow in 1352. The devastation was terrible; historians have reckoned that some 24 million people died, about a quarter of the European population. Crews were entirely wiped out, so that many ships drifted unmanned and helpless about the Mediterranean and North Seas. In southern France mortality was so great that the Pope consecrated the river Rhône at Avignon, so that corpses flung into the river might be considered to have received Christian burial. Both Boccaccio and Petrarch have left horrible descriptions of the plague in Italy. There is an unauthenticated rumour of a small outbreak in England during the late winter of 1347; if true, this must have remained a rat-flea-man infection, for it soon died out.

There is a modern tendency to underestimate the severity of the Black Death. Various reasons are put forward, but the underlying thought is 'it just cannot have happened'. Many people assume that the visitation was little worse than later epidemics. Petrarch appears to have foreseen this attitude. He lived at Avignon in the south of France; his beloved Laura died of the plague in April 1348. Petrarch wrote that future generations would be incredulous, would be unable to imagine the empty houses, abandoned towns, the squalid countryside, the fields littered with dead, the dreadful silent solitude which seemed to hang over the whole world. No one could advise in a time of pestilence such as this; physicians were useless, historians knew of no such visitation, philosophers could only shrug their shoulders and look wise.

Petrarch questioned—and, as it has turned out, rightly questioned—whether posterity could possibly believe such things, when those who had actually seen them could hardly believe them themselves.

The Black Death was not just another incident in the long list of epidemics which have smitten the world. It was probably the greatest European catastrophe in history.

Considering the extent of the disaster, we know surprisingly little of the Black Death; for instance, the very scanty descriptions of signs and symptoms do not so much as mention blood-stained sputum (although *vomiting* of blood is described), yet this is one of the cardinal signs of a virulent pneumonia. Nevertheless, the widespread and high mortality of the plague indicate that it must have been predominantly of the pneumonic type. The English outbreak was brought by ship to the coast of Dorset, where it appeared in the village of Melcombe, now swallowed up in the seaside resort of Weymouth. The usually accepted date is the first week of August 1348, but it has recently been suggested that an infected ship arrived from Gascony shortly before the Feast of St John the Baptist (24 June) and that from this ship 'the men of that town of Melcombe were the first in England to be infected'. Philip Ziegler, who backs this evidence with an extract from the Chronicle of the Grey Friars at Lynn, thinks that a small, local rat-flea-man infection developed at the end of July and that the rapidly spreading pneumonic type appeared in early or middle August.

From the port of Melcombe, the plague travelled both by land and by sea, with coasting vessels bringing infection to ports on the south and west coasts and the Bristol Channel. It then ran quickly north and east through Dorset and Somerset, reaching Bristol by 15 August. It is, however, possible that the infection was brought to Bristol by sea, or even that this may have been a new focus of infection, for Bristol was a port of considerable size and received many ships from Europe. The citizens of Gloucester, learning of the sickness, tried to prevent attack by cutting off all communication with Bristol, but their effort was in vain. From Gloucester the plague passed to Oxford and from Oxford to London, where it first appeared about 1 November. Westward spread, through the relatively sparsely inhabited counties of Devon and Cornwall, was slower, for the plague did not reach Bodmin in central Cornwall until just before Christmas. By then plague was raging throughout the diocese of Bath and Wells, which covered the counties of Dorset and Somerset, for on 4 January 1349 the bishop wrote of a great mortality and of many parishes left without a priest to administer the sacraments.

In London, Parliament was prorogued on 1 January 1349 because of plague and again on 10 March; there were not many deaths at first, but the sickness increased in violence during winter and spring, rising to a peak in April and May, and then gradually declining. The same story is found on the road between Bristol and London, for Oxford was first infected before November 1348 but the time of greatest mortality was not until 1349.

From London the main route lay through the very highly populated eastern counties, Norwich being infected in March 1349 and York on Ascension Day; that is, during the latter part of May. By now the whole of the south, east, and midland districts of England had been attacked and the rate of spread slowed up in the more thinly populated north and west. Ireland received the infection by sea in 1349, but Wales and Scotland were not attacked until 1350. Scotland might quite possibly have escaped, had not the Scots decided to take advantage of England's difficulties by an invasion in the autumn of 1349 when mortality was at its greatest in the extreme northern counties. Plague broke out in the Scottish army encamped near Selkirk, and was dispersed over the country as the soldiers returned to their homes.

This variation in the rate of progress is only to be expected. Not only were villages more thickly clustered in the south, the midlands, and the east, but these regions had formed the main corn-exporting areas of England, served by roads designed for wagon traffic. The great wagon trains had disappeared but, after only fifty years, the roads were still fit for use. Once established, the infection was spread by man as well as by rats, whether from man to man in the pneumonic type, or by plague-infested fleas which were the constant companions of both man and rat. Fear induced flight from a plague-ridden village; flight was both easier and quicker along an open road or over the cleared lands which had once been under corn. In the north and west of England, in Scotland and Wales, the country was more rugged, villages were more widely separated and roads were few; thus flight was more difficult and the rate of spread slower.

We do not know how many people died during this terrible year. There were no bills of mortality, there was no Domesday Book, no census. No man in 1348 was able to estimate large numbers, to strike a gross figure from investigation of a random sample. We do not even know the total population of England in 1347; it has been estimated as low as $3\frac{1}{2}$ million and as high as 5 million. Further, the Black Death did not occur as a single visitation: there were recurrent epidemics on four or five occasions before the end of the fourteenth century. The worst of these was in 1361 when it raged in England, France and Poland, among other countries. The name *Pestis puerorum*, given to this outbreak, provides our first clue, for it suggests the presence of an abnormally high percentage of children in 1361, as would be the case if all age groups had suffered a great mortality thirteen years before.

Another clue is provided by the Poll Tax levied in 1377. Estimates based upon this tax suggest that the population was about 2,070,000. Since the population in 1348 was at least 3,500,000, there must have been a drop of $1\frac{1}{2}$ million in the total population between 1349 and 1377. The population rose steadily between the Norman Conquest and 1348; it also rose steadily from the end of the fourteenth century onwards, until a figure of at least $3\frac{1}{2}$ million was again reached in the middle of the sixteenth century. In both cases, the rise can only have occurred because the live-birth rate outnumbered the death rate. Ordinary disease, including outbreaks of epidemic illness, caused deaths throughout the whole period; just as the normal process of death continued, so did the normal process of birth. Thus the disappearance of 1½ million people between the years 1349 and 1377 can only have been due to an abnormal mortality. Since a large diminution of fecund adults would prevent a rising birth rate, it is safe to assume that maximum mortality occurred at the beginning of the twenty-eight-year period.

There must have been considerable variation in the pattern of infection, and so of mortality, throughout England and Europe. The crowded, walled towns would obviously have been at high risk. Density of population and easy communications conduced to a high rate of infection and the rapid spread of disease. In the thickly populated eastern counties of England, where villages lay cheek by jowl and roads had been maintained for wagon traffic, the death toll must have been large. Inland waterways and coastal traffic would also have favoured spread. In the thinly populated areas of the west and north of Britain, and to a lesser extent in some southern counties, there must have been quite large districts which escaped entirely, simply because of bad communications. But in 1348 the riches and the greater part of the population of England were concentrated in the eastern and midland counties; a high mortality here would have exerted so profound an effect that the relative freedom from disease of wide areas, largely composed of forest and waste, can be almost discounted.

The immediate effect of the Black Death was a general paralysis. Trade largely ceased; the war between England and France was halted by a truce on 2 May 1349 and did not break out again generally until September 1355. In 1350, with the death of so many able-bodied men, the defence of the realm became a matter of grave concern, and towns were required to supply men-at-arms, ships and sailors from their depleted resources.

The cornfields had been sown or were being sown while the plague still gathered momentum. Although a disease of cattle and sheep is mentioned as occurring during the Black Death, there was far greater destruction of men than of livestock. Many more wills were proved during the Black Death than at any time before or for many years to come. For

41

instance, in normal times about three wills per month were probated in the Hustings Court of London; in January to November 1349 the number ranged from eighteen to 121 per month. Those who survived the pestilence encountered unwonted prosperity; there was more money per head, more livestock and more grain. Because it was a buyer's market, prices fell steeply to a third or less of their previous level. A good horse which had been worth forty shillings now fetched only sixteen; a fat ox could be bought for four shillings, a cow for one shilling, a fat sheep for fourpence. Wheat, which had been as cheap as sixteen pence a quarter in the great corn-growing years and as dear as twenty-six shillings in the lean year of 1315-16, was sold at one shilling a quarter.

The urgent need to reap the harvest in the autumn of 1349 induced landowners to offer high wages; in the eastern, mid-land, and southern counties, reapers and mowers received at least double their ordinary wage. The diet of the surviving labourers became unwontedly good as a result of all this plenty. These are the days of which William Langland wrote that Hunger was no longer Master. Beggars refused bread made of beans and demanded milk loaves or fine white wheaten bread and the best brown ale. Day labourers, who had once been content to eat stale vegetables and a hunk of cold bacon washed down with small beer, now turned up their noses at anything except fresh meat and fried or baked fish, served hot lest they catch a chill on their stomachs.

This time of gross plenty was of short duration, for only a limited number of cattle could be tended and only a limited acreage cultivated by the reduced labour force. The Statutes of Labourers, enacted by Parliament in 1350 and 1351 were aimed not only at the labourer. These laws, although they sought to peg wages at the level obtaining in 1346, also directed victuallers and other traders to sell their goods at reasonable prices. This was, in fact, the first example of a Prices and Incomes Policy.

The continuing rise in population until 1347 had out-stripped the land available for cultivation. There was, in fact, a glut of labour. The Black Death reversed this situation. In the years immediately following, shortage of labour was so extreme and disorganization so great in the previously heavily-populated areas that legislation could do nothing to effect a remedy. But those areas less severely affected still possessed an excess of labour in 1350. Thus, given mobility, there was still a small pool of labour available and so wages could be held down. This pool was, however, not sufficiently large to solve the problem in the long term when further plagues and fewer births made labour increasingly scarce. But, at least until 1361, the Statutes of Labourers succeeded in restoring some measure of stability by preventing wages and prices from getting entirely out of control.

During and immediately after the Black Death, the labouring class became mobile for the first time in English history. At first the driving force was the natural urge to escape from pestilence, the instinct of the few survivors of a devastated community to seek their livelihoods elsewhere. Later, in the autumn and winter of 1349, the vital need to gather in the harvest dictated the purposeful mobilization of the available labour force. This movement was local but, as the scarcity of labour became more acute, rumours of higher wages tempted workers to travel further afield and to seek new masters. The masters, although more than willing to enforce the principle of feudal tenure, found themselves so short of labour that they were obliged to hire the vagabonds without questioning their origin.

The Statutes applied not only to the labourer but to his master. Just as the labourer might not demand higher wages, so the master might not offer them. These masters were not always great landlords. Many villeins had become substantial small farmers, cultivating as much as thirty or forty acres. They were not free men, in that they held their land by service to their lords or had commuted that service for a payment in cash or kind. But they were masters in that they employed hired labour, drawn from the landless or almost landless class of 'cottars and bordars' which had greatly increased during the thirteenth century.

The great landlord, already in difficulty in 1349, was faced

43

with a virtually insoluble dilemma after the available labour force had been further decreased in 1361. Many of his service tenants had died and their holdings were back in his hands. If he wished to farm this land himself, he needed labourers. If he did not farm it, the only profitable alternative was to let the land at a rent. The only person willing to rent part of this increased acreage was the surviving villein, whose duty it had been to till and cultivate his lord's fields. The land-owner government attempted to solve the dilemma by enforcing feudal rights without mercy; not only did commutation for payment cease entirely but service was demanded from those who had already commuted.

Obviously this attempted solution created increasing hardship as the available labour declined and, equally obviously, it evoked intense hostility among that section of the labouring community which had already tasted comparative freedom. Hostility increased through twenty troubled years and crystallized in the revolt of 1381. Although precipitated by the unpopular Poll Tax of 1377, this was predominantly an agricultural rising, having as its chief objective commutation of all servile dues for 'a fair rent' of fourpence an acre. The revolt failed in its immediate purpose and was followed by harsh repression but, in the end, the landlord at last understood that his only feasible course was to make the best bargain that he could with his villeins. He retained ownership of the land but ceased to farm that land through his bailiff or reeve. The reeve, who had overseen the labourers on his lord's fields, became the estate steward who received the rents from his lord's tenants. The service-labourer or villein developed into the tenant-farmer. Thus the Black Death struck such a blow to the already weakened feudal system that it had lost much of its meaning within two generations and had entirely disappeared within 150 years. But the tenant-farmer himself needed hired labour; this he drew from the less able villein and from the landless class of cottar and bordar. The new pattern had become evident by the early years of the fifteenth century and was complete in the sixteenth: England had become a country of tenant-farmers,

44

their fields worked by a landless agricultural proletariat. In the majority of European countries the feudal system lingered on for four or five centuries, but in England the peasant ceased to exist; farmer and landworker took his place.

The new tenant-farmer lived closer to the soil than the old aristocratic landlord-cultivator. He understood more readily than his late master that an excessive acreage can only be economically farmed by methods which require a small labour force. Thus he quickly decreased the area of arable and increased his pasture. Even in the strong corn-growing lands of East Anglia, sheep became the farm staple; in the north and west, sheep virtually ousted all other crops. Tudor prosperity depended upon wool. So rapid was the change that shortage of labour had again turned to glut in the fifteenth century and, by the time of Henry VIII, the complaint was heard that the sheep were eating up the men. We catch a glimpse of the starving, out-of-work ploughman and reaper in the often-misquoted nursery rhyme:

> *Baa baa, black sheep, have you any wool?*
> *Yes sir, no sir, three bags full.*
> Two *for my master and* one *for his dame*
> *But* none *for the little boy who cries down the lane.*

Thus, within little over a century, the villein-farmer developed into the wool baron. He was helped by the ever-increasing strain imposed upon the landed class by nearly 150 years of more or less continuous warfare. But, had it not been for the labour crisis that followed the Black Death, the ex-villein would never have been able to take advantage of the anarchy that accompanied the Wars of the Roses. In the dynastic struggle of 1455-61 the old feudal aristocracy of England committed mass suicide and the late villein, now tenant-farmer, emerged as the landowner, by buying up the estate of his ruined lord. The large majority of older English 'county families' arose during this time and by this means; their origins lie in a Saxon and villein ancestry rather than in Norman blood. These 'new men' came to power under

45

the Tudors. Unlike the Norman barons, the 'new men' were of the same stock as their inferiors; though sometimes harsh and arrogant and often bitterly resented, they never developed into a closed, aloof caste like the Continental aristocracy. The strength of the English social structure lies in this fact; continuing shifts have prevented a rigid differentiation between classes.

Petrarch must be right. No man who has not lived through a great and incurable plague can possibly imagine the horror and despair that attend it. Appeals to human aid and divine intervention are alike in vain. The Black Death must have seemed to be of supernatural origin, a punishment inflicted by a higher power upon unknown sinners for unknown crimes. Culprits were sought: nobles, cripples, and Jews in turn came under suspicion. The Jews, in particular, were suspected of purposely spreading plague by contaminating wells or by 'anointing' houses and persons with an imagined poison. Their persecution started at Chillon on Lake Geneva in 1348 and rapidly spread to Basel, Bern, Freiburg and Strassburg. At Basel and Freiburg all known Jews were herded into a large wooden building and burned to death. At Strassburg over two thousand are said to have been hanged on a scaffold set up in the Jewish burial ground. So bitter did the persecution become that the liberal Pope Clement VI issued two Bulls declaring Jews to be innocent. Numbers fled from western Europe into east Germany and Poland. Here they were tolerated and founded communities which rapidly grew in numbers, a fact which helps to account for the very large Jewish population of west Russia, eastern Germany, Poland, and north-east Austria in the nineteenth and early twentieth centuries. Thus the Black Death intensified the mediaeval Christian tradition of the scapegoat-Jew and, by causing the migration of so large a number to the east and north of Europe, is linked to the pogroms of Imperial Russia and the gas-chambers of Auschwitz.

The attempt to find a culprit was accompanied, on the one hand, by a general relaxation of moral values and a cynical, unhappy pursuit of pleasure. On the other hand, there developed a masochistic urge to accept or divert the divine punishment. The most dramatic expression of this urge was the mania for organized mass flagellation. The flagellants were not a product of the Black Death alone, for they rose to some notoriety in Italy and Germany following a severe famine-pestilence in 1258-9. But in 1348 the movement spread all over Europe and enlisted tens of thousands. The flagellants organized themselves in companies each under a master, wore a special uniform, lived under discipline, and conducted their public and private self-flagellations according to a set ritual. To our minds the flagellants are extraordinary and rather horrible, but the reason for their strange behaviour is perfectly logical: the Black Death was a divine chastisement; the flagellant attempted to divert the divine punishment by chastising himself. Thus it was the rumour rather than the appearance of plague which induced the exhibition; the flagellant tried to forestall punishment of his fellows by inflicting punishment upon his own body.

The movement was at first welcomed by the Church as a mass penance. Pope Clement himself ordered public flagellation at Avignon in an attempt to stay the plague. But the flagellants rapidly got out of control and assumed the character of a revolutionary movement directed against Jews, the richer classes and the Church alike. In October 1349 the Pope issued a Bull against them. Many were beheaded, hanged, or burned, and all further processions were forbidden. A curious quirk of clerical psychology condemned a number of flagellants to be flogged by priests before the high altar of St Peter's in Rome.

The Christian Church had risen to be a dominant power partly as a result of the earlier pestilences. It would be strange if so great a catastrophe as the Black Death did not exert some influence upon the authority of a religion which had now been established for 1,000 years. The remarkable grasp of the Church upon Europe enabled Christianity to weather the storm, but the authority of the Church did not survive the Black Death unscathed.

Up to a point, Church influence had been for the public good; she preserved a limited peace in times of strife, tried to impose a code of human behaviour, and acted as schoolmistress. The Church harnessed and nourished intellect, taught and provided administrators, lawyers and physicians, encouraged and preserved architecture, literature and art. But, although creative work might be encouraged, creative thought was more often sternly repressed. The doctrine of persecution formed an integral part of mediaeval Christianity and those whose written or spoken thoughts did not follow the rigid line permitted by the Church stood in danger of persecution as heretics.

In material matters the Church suffered badly from the Black Death. A great loss of manpower and impoverishment through inability to cultivate her vast tracts of land rendered her a less dominant power in 1350 than in 1346. But greater harm resulted from her helplessness in this time of disaster, a large loss of priests and monks, and her failure to control their successors. Parish priests, the best-loved of church workers, died by the hundred and according to William Langland their benefices were all too often hurriedly filled by 'numbers of youths, that had only devoted themselves for clerks by being shaven'. If Langland is to be believed—and there is no reason to disbelieve him—the friars, who had previously been renowned for holiness and charity, gave themselves up to 'gayness and gluttony', while country parsons and parish priests spent their time in London, touting for high places, instead of ministering to their parishioners. Langland specifically states in both instances that these abuses had multiplied 'sithen the pestilence time'.

Further, the very fact that the Church possessed the seeming advantage of being international or supra-national implied a threat to her power. In many countries, Germany and England for example, People and Church had been falling out of sympathy for a number of years. The national branches of the Church cried out for reform, but they had no power to reform themselves because they lacked autonomy; they were, in fact, outlying parts of a foreign organization of immense power and prestige.

For all these reasons, open opposition to the Church developed in the years immediately following the Black Death. Popular reaction can be measured by contrasting the murders of two prominent English churchmen. In 1170 the Archbishop of Canterbury was done to death as the result of some hasty words spoken by King Henry II; although Thomas à Becket's policy was not generally approved, public horror at this sacrilege forced the king to submit himself to humiliating penance. In 1381 a band of rebels seized the mild Simon Sudbury, Archbishop of Canterbury, and struck off his head on Tower Hill in London amid the ferocious applause of a great crowd. 'The relation of Church and people had undergone a profound change since the ancestors of these same men had knelt beside their ploughs to pray for the Holy Martyr, Thomas à Becket,' wrote G. M. Trevelyan.

The change was more profound than is suggested by the murder of Sudbury, Langland's disapproval or the deviant behaviour of flagellants. John Wyclif, born about 1320 and dying in 1384, was a notable theologian and Master of Balliol College, Oxford. He questioned Holy Church's hitherto unchallenged power. As well as demanding a vernacular Order of Service and translating the Bible into English, he attacked the worship of images and relics, the sale of pardons and masses for the dead. Wyclif gained an immense following who became known as the Lollards. They were drawn not only from the common people, but from the friars and some of the lesser clergy who had reason to dislike wealthy monks and bishops.

Wyclif was before his time. As the Church re-established its shaken authority, the Lollards became subject to persecution and were driven underground, to reappear in the reigns of Henry VII and VIII. Persecuted again, they re-emerged to combine with the Protestants of Martin Luther. Luther owed something to the teaching of the earlier reformer John Huss of Bohemia, and Huss, in turn, acknowledged himself a pupil of Wyclif. Thus it is not too much to claim that the

Protestant Reformation, the sailing of the Brownist Pilgrim Fathers in the *Mayflower* from Plymouth on 6 September 1620 and the foundation of Pennsylvania by the Quaker William Penn in 1681, can all be linked with the deviation from established religion that followed the disaster of the Black Death.

One would have thought that so great a pestilence, in which physicians and priests alike proved useless, must have profoundly affected the development of the theocratic medical art. This is not so. Almost the only medical advance directly attributable to the Black Death is in the field of public health. In 1374 the Venetian republic appointed three officials whose duty was to inspect and to exclude all infected vessels from the ports. In 1377 Ragusa detained travellers from infected places for thirty days (*trentini giorni*). When this proved ineffective, the period of detention was lengthened to forty days (*quaranti giorni*); from this early preventive measure comes our modern word 'quarantine'.

Besides this, the Black Death added yet another saint to the Calendar. St Roch is the special patron of bubonic plague. A native of Montpellier, he nursed the sick during the Black Death in north Italy and himself fell a victim. Left to die, Roch was succoured by a dog and recovered. He returned to his home town but was suspected of being a spy and cast into prison, where he died. Here again is the pattern of mortal hurt, miraculous recovery, and ultimate death.

We should honour the Church for her unremitting care of the sick, but acknowledge that her influence upon medical and scientific advance was almost wholly evil. The 1,000-year repression of many forms of creative thought between the fall of Rome and the Renaissance provides a miserable picture of sterile plagiarism. Great schools of medicine were founded—Salerno and Bologna in Italy, Paris and Montpellier in France—but the teaching in those schools was an uncritical reiteration of ancient theories, and research took the form of disputations upon the exact meaning of a text. The vast medical literature of this long period contains many original observations but scarcely any original thought; it is little better than a series of compilations, the substance derived from Latin texts of first-century authors and their Islamic commentators. There are, of course, occasional flashes of the divine fire, for no weight of repression will ever stifle criticism entirely. Thus Mundinus of Bologna defied the ban upon human dissection and did something to restore the science of anatomy to the standard reached by Greek workers about 300 B.C. Another flame in the darkness is Roger Bacon of Oxford and Paris, a philosopher rather than a physician and certainly an original thinker, but his originality earned him imprisonment for the last thirteen years of his life.

The habit of thought engendered by theocratic intolerance stifled medical advance until the end of the fifteenth century. Galen remained the unquestioned authority. This dominance of one man would have been bad enough in itself, but the texts of Galen had been so debased as to be almost worthless. The true teachings of Galen were not restored until too late when, at the end of the fifteenth century, a new way of thinking opened up great vistas of learning and beauty. The wonderful phenomenon of the Renaissance was not merely a revival of classical culture; it was a change in the whole outlook of thinking men, who demanded escape from the tyranny of dogmatism, from the limitations of thought imposed by the Church. Although the ghost of Galen was not laid until William Harvey disproved his doctrine of the ebb-and-flow movement of blood in the seventeenth century, it was the Renaissance that finally broke the Church's stranglehold upon medicine.

Bubonic plague remained one of the more lethal European diseases for three centuries after the Black Death. It disappeared from the greater part of Europe during the early years of the eighteenth century, but remained endemic on the southern and eastern shores of the Mediterranean, in Asia, in Africa and in South America; epidemics have reached the proportion of national pandemics at times. A great outbreak in Manchuria during 1910-11 was almost entirely of the pneumonic type and must have resembled the Black Death. European travellers to infected regions can still become infected.

Prevention and treatment of bubonic plague are now reasonably successful. The causative organism, *Pasteurella pestis*, was discovered almost simultaneously by a Japanese, Shiramiro Kitasato, and a Swiss, Alexander Yersin, during an outbreak at Hong Kong in 1884. Prevention was found to be possible by inoculation with a killed vaccine or by injection of a live avirulent organism, that is, a relatively harmless strain of *Pasteurella pestis*. Antibiotic drugs, streptomycin or tetracyclin, give good results when administered to infected patients. One of the more important preventive measures is control of rats and fleas. Rats can be killed by Warfarin; fleas by one of the persistent insecticides such as Dicophane (DDT) or benzene hexachloride (BHC). But bubonic plague, especially of the pneumonic type, is still so dangerous that sick attendants must wear masks, protective gowns and gloves, just as they did or were advised to do in the Black Death and the Great Plague of 1665.

But the success of modern measures does not explain why plague disappeared from Europe in the eighteenth century. Here is one of the mysteries of medicine. The answer cannot be a mass resistance as is the case with some other diseases, for plague resembles a cold in that little immunity is conferred by one attack. Nor, as is sometimes suggested, can the Great Fire of London have had any influence, for the effect of rebuilding in brick could only have been local. The 'rat theory' at first sounds more hopeful. The black rat has almost disappeared from inland Europe, exterminated by the stronger and more ferocious brown rat. The black rat, companionable with man, is more likely to infect him with plague-bearing fleas. The brown rat can also become infected with *Pasteurella pestis* and does carry fleas, but is not companionable with man and so the chances of rat-flea-man spread are greatly lessened. The 'rat theory' might therefore account for the disappearance of plague provided that it could be shown that the brown rat replaced the black rat at the end of the seventeenth century. But in England, plague virtually disappeared after 1666; the brown rat did not arrive until 1728. As late as 1783, the black was the commoner species in London, Middlesex, and Buckinghamshire. It is possible, however, that the slow spread of the brown rat across Europe in the early eighteenth century may have upset a symbiotic mechanism.

The question of why this one particular infection vanished from Europe at the time that it did really remains unanswered. Perhaps the Black Death has not disappeared but gone into hiding, as it seems to have done between the sixth and the fourteenth centuries. If this is so, there may yet be unpleasant surprises in store for us.

3
The Mystery of
Syphilis

One of the most controversial problems in medical history is the question of how and why syphilis suddenly emerged in Europe at the end of the fifteenth century. Syphilis is now primarily a venereal disease, spreading from person to person by direct contact during sexual intercourse. But syphilis can also be acquired innocently by sharing a drinking vessel or by infection through a wound. After the initial infection there follows an incubation period of from ten to ninety days, usually two to four weeks, before the first signs of disease appear. The first sign takes the form of a chancre, the local tissue reaction to inoculation, which is an ulcer found at the site of contact. Obviously, the chancre will usually develop on or around the genital organs, but it may occur at any place when the disease has been innocently acquired. The chancre, even when untreated, will often disappear spontaneously within three to eight weeks, leaving a very thin and inconspicuous scar. Sometimes it is quite large and sometimes little more than a rather hard pimple. About a quarter of all patients seen at the special clinics deny that they have noticed this primary lesion.

Six to eight weeks after the appearance of the chancre, the patient will develop symptoms of a secondary stage, but these symptoms are sometimes delayed for a year or even more. The secondary stage is a general tissue reaction to the infection. It is much like any reaction to bacterial invasion. There is a feeling of discomfort, headache, perhaps sore throat, a mild fever and, in about 75 per cent of cases, a skin rash. This rash is rather important in our story, because it may take a number of forms. Syphilis is known as 'the great mimic' because it can be mistaken on superficial examination for so many other diseases. This is particularly true of the rash, which sometimes bears a resemblance to measles, smallpox, or one of many skin diseases. As a rule this secondary stage does not last for long and the patient then enters an early latent stage, in which he appears entirely free of all signs and symptoms, although sometimes his rash will reappear for a time and then disappear again. During both the secondary active and early latent stages the patient is highly infectious; the really dangerous period is during the early latent stage, for he is able to infect others but himself appears to be quite free from infection.

After about two years there develops a late latent stage, in which there are no signs or symptoms and the patient is often not capable of passing on the disease. It cannot be said that he is cured, because blood tests will reveal the presence of syphilis in his tissues, but the disease is quiescent and may remain so for the rest of the patient's life span, death occurring from some unrelated cause. This is a quite common event even if the syphilis is untreated.

It is for this reason that syphilis is so dangerous. The late latent stage may last for years without incident, the patient living in a fool's paradise believing that he will encounter no further trouble. But he is often wrong, for the disease has only settled into a very chronic phase. From three to ten years after the primary infection, but often at an even later date, the signs of tertiary syphilis may appear. There are many manifestations, for syphilis can attack almost every system in the body. The typical lesion, the gumma, can appear anywhere—in the bones, the heart, the throat, the skin. Tertiary syphilis may be shown by changes in the blood-vessels, resulting in weakening and ballooning of the walls, which leads to death by rupture of the aorta or one of the vessels of the brain. The nervous system can be affected, causing the condition known as tabes dorsalis when the patient gradually becomes paralysed and incontinent. Or the brain itself may be damaged, giving rise to horrible person-ality changes and sometimes ending in general paralysis of the insane (GPI), in which the sufferer is converted into a helpless maniac. Often this latter state is presaged by a phase in which the patient has ideas or schemes that are rational but unusual or grandiose. Conan Doyle tells the story of a young farmer who surprised all his neighbours by taking a very rosy view of farming prospects during a time of depres-sion. He proposed to give up orthodox cropping and to corner the market by planting the whole of his farm with rhododen-drons. Most untreated patients die within five years of show-ing the first signs of GPI, but a number never become frankly insane or helpless; the disease process in the brain changes their pattern of behaviour but they are able to carry on more or less normal lives and die from some other illness. The usual symptoms of tertiary syphilis affecting the nervous system are headache, lightning pains, impotence, adult epilepsy, and an apoplectic stroke at less than fifty years of age. Common signs of commencing GPI are painful joints, neurasthenia and character changes.

One of the more terrible attributes of syphilis is that it can be transmitted from parent to child. If the mother is in the active stage, her child will probably die while still unborn; death does not usually occur until the fourth month of pregnancy at the earliest. Thus it can be stated that a history of repeated miscarriages *before* the fourth month of pregnancy is not suggestive of syphilis, but that repeated miscarriages *after* the fourth month are strongly suggestive. As the mother passes through the later stages, the child will have a better chance of being born alive; finally, when and if the disease has cured itself spontaneously, normal healthy children may be born. A 'typical' pattern of births would run as follows:

First pregnancy	Miscarriage at fifth month.
Second pregnancy	Stillbirth at eighth month.
Third pregnancy	Live, but dies of syphilis soon after birth.
Fourth pregnancy	Live, showing signs of syphilis weeks or months after birth.
Fifth pregnancy	Apparently healthy child, showing signs of syphilis after a few years.
Sixth pregnancy	Child healthy until his teens, then showing signs of syphilis.
Seventh pregnancy	Healthy child, never showing signs of syphilis.

But syphilis only rarely produces a 'typical pattern' and healthy children may alternate with diseased children in a syphilitic family.

The diseased children develop the disease through the same stages as the adult. But, because the disease process is affecting a growing individual, some special signs are often, though not always, present. These include bone defects, impaired sight and hearing, and deformed teeth. The well-known 'Hutchinson's Triad', first described by Jonathan Hutchinson of the London Hospital in 1861, consists of deafness, impaired vision, and notched, peg-shaped teeth. The deafness is caused by damage to the auditory nerve. The particular defect of vision is known as interstitial keratitis, which first appears as a diffuse haziness near the centre of one cornea and occurs most commonly between the ages of five and fifteen. The haziness spreads over the cornea and the other eye is attacked two or three months later. The child goes temporarily blind, or almost blind, but a surprising improvement occurs within a year or eighteen months. Patches of haze often remain for life, so that vision may never be entirely normal. For some unknown reason, almost twice as many male children are affected. They suffer eye pain in strong light and often develop a habit of lowering the eyelids and eyebrows as though frowning.

In considering the history of syphilis, it is important to remember that everything said above refers to the untreated disease of today. It does not necessarily follow that exactly the same clinical picture was observed by physicians when syphilis first made its appearance in Europe at the end of the fifteenth century.

From 1490 onwards something which appeared to contemporary writers to be a new disease swept over Europe. Thence it spread to India, China, Japan and, eventually, to the rest of the world. Early medical historians accepted that this new disease originated in the army of Charles VIII who, having launched an invasion of Italy in the autumn of 1494, attacked Naples in February 1495, or that it started in the city and was transmitted to the French army. This army of about 30,000 men was not, in fact, French but was composed of mercenary troops, French, German, Swiss, English, Hungarian, Polish and Spanish. The great number of sick forced Charles to withdraw and abandon his attempted conquest of northern Italy. This, at least, is fact and provides us with an example of how disease can affect the course of history. The classical story—or perhaps legend—continues that the remnant of Charles's disbanded army streamed back to their homes, thus spreading the disease throughout the many parts of Europe from which they came. Very shortly afterwards the sickness became known by names which varied according to the supposed country of origin. We hear of 'the Neapolitan', 'the French' and 'the Polish' disease. Later it became known in China as 'Canton disease' and in Japan as 'the Chinese disease'. Englishmen knew it as 'the French pox' or 'the great pox'; in France it was often called *la grosse vérole*. The French also named it 'the Spanish disease' and this brings us to the earliest theory of the origin of syphilis.

Christopher Columbus first saw the New World, probably one of the Bahama Islands, on 12 October 1492. Between October and January he visited Cuba and Haiti. In the latter month he set sail for Europe, landing at Palos, the port from which he had set out, on 15 March 1493. He brought with him ten natives from the West Indies, of whom one died soon after landing, and a crew of forty-four men. The crew were disbanded and some are said to have joined the troops of Gonzalo de Cordoba who marched with Charles VIII to Naples. Columbus travelled with his nine natives to Seville, left three of them there, and took the remaining six on to Barcelona. At the end of April the six Indians, all males, were shown naked to the court; they are described as brown and comely, more like Asiatics than Africans. There is no mention of any disease.

Twenty-five years later, in 1518, a book, printed in Venice, first mentioned the theory that a 'Spanish disease' had been imported from America (or the West Indies) by seamen in the 1492-3 expedition led by Columbus. This theory was supported and popularized in 1526 by Gonzalo Fernandez de Oviedo y Valdes, who had been a page at the Spanish court when Columbus showed his Indians. Oviedo made several voyages to the West Indies and reported that he had found evidence of the new disease among the natives. In 1539 Rodrigo Ruiz Diaz de Isla, a physician, published a description of 'the West Indian disease' or *bubas*', and claimed to have treated at least one, if not more, of Columbus's crew at Barcelona. Diaz de Isla practised in several of the larger Spanish ports, so he may, after a lapse of over forty years, have written Barcelona in mistake for Palos or Lisbon.

The first theory therefore maintains that syphilis was introduced into Europe from the West Indies by ship in 1493. Many medical historians support this opinion. The evidence in favour is that a new disease of great virulence undoubtedly did appear in Europe at about the time of Columbus's return. Another point, sometimes cited, is that one of the earliest and more popular treatments was by holy wood or guaiacum, a resin obtained from two evergreen trees, *Guaiacum officinale* and *Guaiacum sanctum*, which are indigenous to South America and the West Indies. Guaiacum was introduced in 1508, that is, ten years before the first mention of West Indian origin; this, of course, is a point in favour of the theory. But its opponents hold that the useless guaiacum was imported not because it was a traditional remedy, but deliberately to support the theory of West Indian origin. Also against the theory must be set the fact that there is no evidence whatsoever of disease in the imported Indians or among the forty-four seamen who returned with Columbus; the homeward voyage seems to have been remarkably healthy. It may, too, be of some significance that the Columban or American theory did not achieve any popularity until over a quarter of a century after his return and the alleged first appearance of the disease. There is, of course, always the possibility that new facts may have come to light in later expeditions to the Indies.

The second theory holds that syphilis originated in Africa and was introduced into Spain and Portugal by the importation of slaves. There is an African disease, yaws, which is bacteriologically indistinguishable from syphilis but which, unlike the modern infection, is chiefly transmitted by non-venereal contact. It is particularly common among children who play together naked. For this reason yaws is seen only in hot climates, where it appears as a horrible skin eruption. The causative organism is the same as that of syphilis; if introduced into cold climates, where people are customarily fully clothed, yaws will settle down into ordinary syphilis, carried mainly by venereal contact. In fact, yaws and syphilis are probably different manifestations of one and the same disease. If it be allowed that early sixteenth century syphilis was a yaws-like disease, as it seems to have been, then there is evidence which suggests that it was brought to Europe from Africa.

In 1442 a Portuguese expedition, led by Prince Henry the Navigator, explored the Atlantic coast of Africa and anchored in the Bight of Benin. One of the captains, Autam Gonçalves, captured a few Moors and took them as prisoners on board his ship. Prince Henry ordered Gonçalves to return them. This he did; the Moors' friends rewarded him with some gold dust and ten African Negroes. The Negroes fetched a large price in Portugal and led to a quite extensive trade in Negro slaves from Africa to Portugal and Spain. The descendants of many of these slaves became Christians. In 1502 King Ferdinand ordered that Christian slaves, particularly from the districts around Seville, should be shipped to the West Indies. So many were sent that the governor of Haiti became alarmed at the number of Negroes in the island and in 1503 asked that transport of slaves should cease.

The suggestion is that these Negro slaves brought yaws with them from Africa and that yaws became syphilis when it infected the fully clothed Portuguese and Spaniards. This theory is a very attractive one and explains much that has gone before; it will also explain much that follows. The Columban or American theory can be made to fit in, for the suggestion of an American origin was first published in 1518; that is, sixteen years after the first African slaves had been sent to the West Indies. But obvious skin disease, often confused with leprosy, aroused particular horror in our forefathers. It has been sensibly argued that the six Indians brought back by Columbus cannot have been diseased, for someone would surely have noticed a skin lesion when they were shown naked at court. But the same argument could be applied to African slaves; in view of the general fear of skin diseases, traders would hardly have shipped Negroes who suffered from yaws.

An extension of the African theory of origin places the introduction of syphilis to Europe at a much earlier date. Equatorial African Negroes found their way to Egypt, Arabia, Greece and Rome; they may have brought yaws with them. This implies that syphilis is a very old disease in Europe and that something unknown caused a flare-up at the end of the fifteenth century. Some historians hold that leprosy, often said to have been brought back from the Levant by crusaders, was in fact syphilis. It is undoubtedly true that leprosy disappeared from Europe or from medical literature and that syphilis took its place. It is also true that both these diseases can produce horrible skin eruptions.

One objection to this theory of an ancient origin is that syphilis not infrequently causes permanent and visible changes in the bones, yet no evidence of syphilitic disease has ever been found in European bones which can be placed at an earlier date than the fifteenth century. Another objection is that our forefathers had no doubt that a new disease of great virulence spread fairly rapidly over Europe in the 1490s. They possessed none of our modern aids to diagnosis and their descriptions are not always as clear as we should wish, but they were capable of honest observation.

What was the nature of this disease which appeared during the fifteenth century and received so many names—great pox or French pox in England, *grosse vérole* in France, *bubas* in Spain? Ulrich von Hutten in 1519 spoke of disgusting sores when the disease first appeared in Germany. He said that after about seven years the disease underwent a change; this acute, obvious skin manifestation became less common and, in consequence, the risk of acquiring infection became greater. Von Hutten made the important observation that at the time of writing in 1519 transmission was by venereal contact. Diaz de Isla, in his description of the disease (1539) described the stages of syphilis as they are known today, but he added a terminal stage of fever, emaciation, diarrhoea, jaundice, abdominal distension, delirium, coma and death. This sounds rather like the syphilitic 'rupia' quite commonly seen a century ago. A modern writer describes rupia as a pustular eruption with extensive destruction of tissue, generally occurring on the face, and causing death from toxaemia.

The most important early work on syphilis was that of Girolamo Frascatoro in 1546. Sixteen years earlier Frascatoro had published at Verona a long poem which he entitled *Syphilis sive Morbus Gallicus*; thus he gave the disease its modern name (derived from an imaginary shepherd Syphilus), although the term did not come into popular use until the end of the eighteenth century. In his very important book of 1546, published at Venice and entitled *De Contagione et Contagiosis Morbis*, Frascatoro examined many diseases which we should now call infectious or contagious. He described syphilis as commencing with small intractable ulcers on the genital organs; the skin then became covered with a pustular rash which usually began on the scalp. These pustules ulcerated to such a depth that bone might be exposed. There was also a 'pernicious catarrh' which eroded the palate, uvula, and pharynx. Sometimes the lips or eyes were entirely eaten away. Later, swellings which he called gummata appeared; these were accompanied by violent pains in the muscles, by lassitude, and by emaciation. Frascatoro was of the opinion that the disease had changed its character in the past twenty years (i.e. since 1526), for he thought that fewer pustules and more gummata were seen at the time of writing.

This virulent new disease did not spread with the speed of bubonic plague. Even if we take 1493 as the date of the first appearance of a syphilis-like disease in Europe, there was a lapse of three years before the invasion of England in 1496. Poland was affected in 1499, Russia and Scandinavia in 1500, and Canton in 1505. Some countries escaped infection until much later: Japan until 1569, Iceland until 1753, while the Faroe Islands were free until as late as 1845. The infection of India in 1498 is of particular historical interest. At first sight this date, only two years after England and one year after Poland, is impossible. The answer is that the crew of the expedition led by Vasco da Gama carried the disease with them from Portugal by the sea route around the Cape of Good Hope to the town of Calicut on the Malabar River, where they landed on 20 May 1498.

In the opening phase of its history, the disease was far more contagious than is the syphilis of today. About a third of the citizens of Paris are said to have become infected. Erasmus wrote that any nobleman who had not had syphilis was considered *'ignobilis et rusticans'*. Very interesting confirmation of the early virulence and later recession is supplied by Sir Thomas More, surely a reliable witness. In 1529 he wrote the tract *Supplication of Souls in Purgatory* in answer to a demand for the suppression of monastic hospitals by Simon Fish. More's tract contains the sentence: 'And then of the french pockes thirty years ago went there about five against one that beggeth with them now.' That is, five patients suffering from syphilis attended the hospitals in 1499 for every one that attended in 1529. If we append to this the statement in 1579 of the London surgeon William Clowes that it is seldom that less than fifteen out of every twenty patients admitted to St Bartholomew's Hospital are suffering from syphilis, then it is clear that the disease must have been very common in the London of 1500.

But why was syphilis so contagious in the early sixteenth century? Part of the answer is supplied if we accept the theory that the disease originated in the African analogue of syphilis called yaws. This would also account for the repeated records of gross skin involvement, for yaws is typically a skin disease. Yaws was going through a transitional phase from the cutaneous non-venereal state to the syphilis of today. The remainder of the answer may lie in a simple fact which has been unaccountably overlooked by all historians of syphilis. The common method of greeting in Tudor times was not the handshake but the kiss.

The more common mode of transmission may have been innocent, that is non-venereal. The disease was passed from one person to another by mouth-to-mouth contact or by drinking from the same vessel. In such cases the primary chancre would have appeared upon the lips or tongue and, in those days of neglected personal hygiene must often have passed unnoticed or have been mistaken for impetigo or herpes (cold sores). Cardinal Wolsey, for instance, was accused of infecting Henry VIII with syphilis by breathing on him. He may have done so but, equally, he may have been suffering from sores on his lips, the result of a severe cold. There must have been many cases of venereal infection, but we need

64

not search for immoral relationships or unsavoury scandals when investigating the syphilis of the early sixteenth century; there is an equal chance that transmission was by innocent contact.

Another reason for the wide spread of syphilis is that the tertiary stage of nervous or arterial involvement was not recognized as being associated with the disease. The gross cutaneous manifestations were not invariably present, and the minor lesions of the early stages—the primary chancre and the secondary rash—could be mistaken for trivial disorders and, in any case, soon disappeared. We have confirmation of this supposition in the dates at which certain terms were first used. The *Oxford English Dictionary* gives the following: Pox 1476, Great Pox 1503, Small Pox 1518. The history of the disease now known as smallpox is obscure; sixteenth-century physicians confused smallpox with measles and regarded the latter as the more dangerous infection. In view of this fact and the dating of the terms, it is possible that Great Pox referred to the major cutaneous manifestation of syphilis more commonly seen in the early years, while Small Pox referred to the secondary rash, more often seen when the disease had lost its initial virulence. In fact 'small pox' may have meant exactly what the name implies, a lesser form of the great pox. For these reasons we must suppose that many infected people went through life untreated, and without even realizing that they suffered from the disease.

The effects of syphilis have been devastating. The tale of suffering and misery is never-ending. A quite random review shows that this foul disease has caused the deaths or—worse—wrecked the lives of the following: among rulers, Charles VIII and Francis I of France; among clerics, Pope Alexander Borgia, his nephew Peter Borgia, and his major-domo the Cardinal-Bishop of Segovia; among artists, Benvenuto Cellini and Toulouse-Lautrec; among writers and poets, Heinrich Heine, Jules de Goncourt, Alphonse Daudet and Guy de Maupassant. Millions of lesser men have suffered equally. Millions more have suffered indirectly, as we can well see in the history of Ivan the Terrible.

Ivan IV, Grand Duke of Muscovy and first Tsar of All the Russians, was born on 25 August 1530, and ascended the grand-ducal throne when three years old, on the death of his father, Vassili III, in December 1533. Threatened and neglected as a child, he seized power at the early age of fourteen. Outwardly Ivan was a typical Russian prince of his time, spending his next years in hunting, womanizing, drinking, robbing merchants, and terrorizing the unfortunate peasantry. But there was a little more to him; beneath this surface there lay a serious scholar who preferred the company of low-born but educated clerks to that of his illiterate nobles. He chose one of the former, Alexei Ardatchev, as his most intimate adviser. On 16 January 1547 Ivan was crowned Tsar, the first Muscovite ruler to be so styled formally, basing his claim on his descent from Vladimir, grandson of the Byzantine Caesar, Constantine Monomakh. Two weeks later he married a pious and humane woman, Anastasia Zakharina-Koshkina.

In the same year a great fire destroyed almost the whole of Moscow. The Metropolitan (Archbishop) Makary took the opportunity to impress upon Ivan the sinful follies of his youth. There now opened a reign which seemed to be potentially one of the most enlightened in the history of Russia. Some kind of legal code was established; the most oppressive nobles were banished; the all-powerful Church was partially reformed; a few schools were founded in Moscow and the larger cities. Although neither a brave man nor a good general, Ivan inspired his troops with a crusading spirit, captured Kazan from the Tartar horde, and extended his empire down the Volga to the port of Astrakhan. In 1558 he turned westward against the Teutonic Knights and, by the summer of 1560, had reached Riga on the borders of Prussia.

By our standards, Ivan was no doubt a cruel despot even during these early years. By contemporary Russian and indeed European standards, he ruled wisely from 1551 to 1560. He played a vigorous part in the deliberations of his council, but allowed freedom of speech and opinion. He received petitions from all classes of his subjects: for the first and the last time in Russian history, the poorest man in the country could gain access to his sovereign.

In October 1552 Anastasia gave birth to a child, Dmitri, who died when six months old. Nine months later she bore another son, Ivan, and a third, Fedor, in 1558. Probably Tsar Ivan had been infected with syphilis before his marriage. We may surmise—it is only surmise—that the infant Dmitri died of congenital syphilis. Giles Fletcher in *The Russe Commonwealth* described Fedor, who survived Ivan the Terrible, as

> ...of mean stature, somewhat low and gross, of a sallow complexion, and inclining to the dropsy, hawk nosed, unsteady in his pace by reason of some weakness in his limbs, heavy and inactive, yet commonly smiling almost to laughter. For quality otherwise simple and slow witted.

He, too, was probably a congenital syphilitic.

Anastasia died in July 1560. Ivan was quite genuinely broken-hearted and he drowned his grief in a prolonged drunken debauch which started immediately after her funeral. His brain conceived the fantasy that his friend Alexei Ardatchev and his wise adviser, the monk Sylvester, had contrived Anastasia's death by witchcraft. Both were dismissed and imprisoned. He then put to death Ardatchev's brother, a magnificent soldier, with his twelve-year-old son; next, his friend Maria Magdalena, a widow, and her five children. On 21 August 1561, Ivan married a rich Circassian princess, but this did not stop him making a proposal of marriage to Queen Elizabeth I of England in 1563. In the same year he led an immense army to invade Lithuania. He captured the important trading city of Polotsk and seemed to have the country at his mercy. Then his martial mood passed and he returned to his debauches in Moscow, where the new Tsaritsa had given birth to a son, Vassili, who lived for five weeks.

In December 1564 occurred the first incident which clearly shows that Ivan was now suffering from cerebral syphilis

(GPI). Early in the morning of December 3 a number of sleighs drew up in the Kremlin Square. They were loaded with gold, silver and jewels from the palace, and with the Tsar, his wife and his two sons. Then they drove off, leaving no forwarding address. Ivan's first message home read: 'Unable to brook the treachery by which I was surrounded, I have forsaken the state and taken my way whither God shall direct.'

His bewildered nobles and bishops set out in search. They found him in the village of Alexandrov, a hundred miles north-west of Moscow, and besought him to return. Ivan consented, on condition that he was free to execute any 'traitors' he so desired, to live in a house outside the Kremlin, and to have a personal bodyguard of 1,000 men, the *'opritchina'*. He returned to Moscow on 2 February 1565 and the executions started on 4 February. The *opritchina* was extended to number 6,000 bandits, and the new house became a strange monastery with the married Ivan as abbot. Three hundred of the *opritchina* served as monks, clad in black cassocks over their sables and cloth of gold. The day started with early matins at four in the morning and ended at eight with vespers, Ivan praying with such fervour that his forehead was permanently bruised from his prostrations. These bouts of prayer were relieved by visits to the torture chamber, conveniently situated in the cellars.

The remainder of Ivan's reign is a sickening tale of tortures and floggings, of burnings and boilings, of all manner of hideous deaths. The dreadful vengeance for an alleged conspiracy that he exacted on the city of Novgorod, where for five weeks thousands were flogged to death, roasted over slow fires, or pushed under the ice; the executions at Moscow on 25 July 1570, when Ivan and his son Ivan themselves helped in the ghastly work, when Prince Viskavati was hanged from a gallows and sliced to death with knives while Ivan raped the widow and his son raped the eldest daughter—these are but a few of the known incidents of a reign of terror which lasted from 1565 until 1584. Ivan's madness culminated in the slaughter of his own son and heir, the Tsarevitch Ivan, whom he stabbed to death with his steel-pointed staff in a fit of murderous rage on 19 November 1581. Disappointed in his hopes of marrying Elizabeth of England, Ivan made overtures to her cousin Lady Mary Hastings and, when this offer was declined, announced his willingness to marry any kinswoman of the Queen; despite the fact that he was already married, Ivan seems to have been obsessed with the fantasy of a royal union with England. Elizabeth, probably bearing in mind the fortunes of the Russian company which had been founded under the patronage of Ivan in 1553, caused her envoy to assure him that any one of a dozen of her kinswomen would be happy to marry him. Fortunately for some innocent girl, Ivan died before the project went any further. His last days were horrible, a time of sleeplessness, terror and insanity, surrounded by soothsayers, his only relaxation the fondling of his jewels and discoursing on their curative powers. The cause of death was an apoplectic fit while setting the board for a game of chess.

Thousands of his subjects perished because Ivan suffered from syphilis but, in the long term, the effect of his disease may have been even greater. It is possible that Russian history was radically changed by Ivan's failure to pursue the comparatively liberal, almost benevolent, policy of his opening years. It is problematical whether the whole pattern of Russian Tsardom would have developed in a different fashion, but there might have been, in this first of the Tsars, a semblance of enlightened rule rather than of cruel despotism. The murder of the Tsarevitch probably saved the country from a reign more bloodthirsty than his father's, for Ivan the Terrible trained his son in cruelty and lust. But the murder left the throne to the inheritance of a congenital idiot, Fedor. Incapable of rule, he was first under the tutelage of, and then displaced by, Boris Godunov. Chaos descended on Russia after the death of Boris in April 1605; no semblance of unity was achieved until the election of the first Romanov to the throne in 1613.

No authority has ever seriously doubted that Ivan was syphilitic, although there are no reports of a rash, skin disease, or any form of treatment. The case of his near-contemporary, Henry VIII of England, is more controversial. Many writers have emphatically denied that Henry suffered from syphilis. But these writers cannot agree upon an alternative diagnosis. Professor Shrewsbury decides in favour of gout; Mr N. R. Barrett believes that Henry was 'punch drunk', the result of a serious injury in a tournament; Sir Arthur Macnalty in his book *Henry VIII, a Difficult Patient* dismisses syphilis but leaves the diagnosis open; later he suggested that Henry suffered from a chronic inflammation (osteomyelitis) of the femur, again probably the result of an injury; Professor J. J. Scarisbrick adds to this a diagnosis of varicose veins. In view of all these differing opinions, it seems wise to re-examine the evidence, for, whatever was the nature of the disease, there is no doubt that its effect upon Henry profoundly influenced the future history of the English nation.

First, let it be said that there is not the slightest reason why Henry should not have suffered from *all* the diseases so far mentioned. A sixteenth-century man who lived to the age of fifty-six must have counted himself lucky if he suffered from only one disability, for much illness was untreatable in those days. Henry ate and drank enormously; he took an active part in the noble sport of the day, jousting in the lists, in which he is known to have had two bad accidents; he became grossly obese and varicose veins are often associated with obesity; he probably was concussed at some time and he probably did suffer from gout. But this cannot be adduced as proof that he did not also suffer from syphilis.

As syphilis is so often a congenitally acquired disease, let us first consider Henry's children, of whom he had at least four. The known illegitimate child, Henry Fitzroy, Earl of Richmond, died at the age of seventeen in 1536. Beyond the facts that his portrait suggests untreated adenoids and his terminal illness was a lung infection, nothing definite is recorded. Elizabeth, daughter of Anne Boleyn, died at the great age of sixty-nine in 1603. She was short-sighted and may have had reason to think that she could not bear healthy children. 'The

Queen of Scots is lighter of a fair son and I am but a barren stock,' was her remark on hearing of the birth of the future James VI and I of Scotland and England. There is nothing to indicate syphilis in Elizabeth and Henry Fitzroy.

Mary, daughter of Katherine of Aragon, died aged forty-two in 1558. She was very short-sighted. There is no mention of deafness, but she spoke in a voice 'deep toned and rather masculine, so that when she speaks she is heard some distance off', the type of voice often used by a partially deaf person. Her nose is described as 'rather low and wide'; it is reported that her husband, Philip II of Spain, complained of the foul smell which emanated from it. A flattened bridge of the nose is sometimes seen in congenital syphilitics and there is frequently a foul, purulent discharge.

There is some evidence that Mary suffered from amenorrhoea and the same may be true of Elizabeth if she had reason to believe that she was 'but a barren stock'. As none of the three children of Henry VIII produced a child, the only heir to the throne on the death of Elizabeth was James VI of Scotland, son of Mary, Queen of Scots, by her second husband, Henry Stuart. This raises a most intriguing medico-historical problem. Mary's first husband was the young Francis II of France. At the age of seventeen, Francis developed an acute infection of the ear. The great surgeon Ambroise Paré wished to operate but was not permitted to do so. Francis died from an abscess of the brain. Here is the problem. What would have happened if Francis had not developed the infection or if Paré had drained the abscess successfully? A child of Mary by Francis would have been heir to the thrones of England, Scotland and France. Would the three countries have been united under one crown in 1603? Whatever the answer may be, it is obvious that the sterility of Elizabeth and Mary coupled with the early death of Francis II profoundly affected the history of Europe.

Edward, son of Henry's third wife, Jane Seymour, died rather mysteriously at the age of fifteen. He was not the attractive child of the story books, but a fat, flabby boy, never in good health. Edward records in his diary that he 'fell sicke

71

of the mesels and the smallpockes' in April 1552. To this Sir John Hayward added, 'which breaking kindly from him was thought would prove a means to cleanse his body from such unhealthful humours as occasion long sickness and death'. Here is a possible suggestion that the rash was in fact syphilitic. It did not cleanse his body from unhealthful humours, for he died sixteen months later. His death appears to have been from pulmonary tuberculosis (phthisis) but the illness had features which puzzled his doctors. There was a widely held opinion that Edward met his end from poison administered by a nurse who claimed to have a secret remedy. During the last fortnight of life, a skin eruption appeared over his body, his nails fell off, and the top joints of his fingers and toes became necrotic. There is no mention of acute abdominal pain so poisoning by antimony or arsenic, the two most likely drugs, cannot be confirmed with certainty. The clinical picture can just possibly be attributed to tuberculosis, but fits better with a combination of pulmonary tuberculosis and congenital syphilis, not uncommon among slum-dwelling children of the nineteenth century. While there is nothing definite in Edward's story, a suspicion must remain.

There are no portraits of Henry's offspring showing them with open mouths, so we cannot begin to speculate as to whether or not they had Hutchinson's teeth. There is nothing in any known portrait of Edward or Elizabeth to indicate whether they did or did not suffer from congenital syphilis.

Let us now consider Henry's six wives: Katherine of Aragon (marriage lasted twenty-four years), Anne Boleyn (three years), Jane Seymour (seventeen months), Anne of Cleves (six months), Catherine Howard (two years) and Catherine Parr (four years). The obstetrical histories are fairly well documented, though some detail is arguable. One striking fact stands out. There is no record of any live birth, stillbirth, or miscarriage during the six years of marriage with his last two wives, Catherine Howard and Catherine Parr. Henry was over middle age by sixteenth-century standards but should have been capable of fathering children. If, as historians hold, his marriage policy was dictated by the desire to found a strong Tudor male line, then the inference is that Henry became sterile or impotent when aged about forty-nine. This is probably the strongest evidence of syphilis in his marital history.

Katherine of Aragon, the mother of Queen Mary, gave birth to a male infant who died within a few days, and had at least three stillborn children, all in the seventh to eighth month of pregnancy. Anne Boleyn, mother of Queen Elizabeth I, miscarried at six months, at three and a half months, and of a foetus of unknown age. Jane Seymour could have had only the one child, Edward VI, and there is no evidence that Henry ever cohabited with Anne of Cleves. The obstetric history of the wives must be regarded as rather suspicious although not certainly diagnostic of syphilis.

As for Henry himself, he was described in his youth by the Venetian Pasquiligo as being:

> The handsomest potentate I ever set eyes on: above the usual height, with an extremely fine calf to his leg; his complexion fair and bright, with auburn hair combed straight and short in the French fashion, and a round face so very beautiful that it would become a pretty woman, his throat being rather long and thick.

The nineteen-year-old boy had everything: physical beauty, a magnificent presence, charm, a fine brain. He was perhaps the finest specimen of manhood ever to wear a crown. He revelled in hunting and all sports, in dancing and music, but his chancellor Wolsey makes it plain that Henry also attended to his business of ruling, held strong opinions, and was not easily overborne.

In February 1514, when twenty-three years old, he fell sick of the smallpox; pustules did not develop and he made a seemingly uneventful recovery. In 1521 he had his first attack of malaria, a common enough disease in sixteenth-century England; he suffered intermittently from malaria throughout his life. Three years later, in March 1524, Henry met with an accident while jousting with the Duke of Suffolk, but he does not seem to have sustained a severe injury. In 1527 he started to suffer from headaches and in 1527-8 he developed the notorious ulcer on his thigh (or thighs) which plagued him for the rest of his life.

In 1527, the crucial year, Henry was aged thirty-six. Until then he ruled wisely and with moderation. More than one dangerous riot, for instance the 'evil May Day' of 1517, was put down firmly but without cruelty—by the standards of those days. During these years Henry laid the foundations of the English naval administration, built ships, founded Trinity House, improved harbours, and established shipyards and storehouses. In 1521, aided by 'all the learned men of England', he wrote the scholarly counterblast to Martin Luther which earned him from Pope Leo X the title of Defender of the Faith, used by his successors upon the throne until the present day. He encouraged Thomas More in his efforts to provide a clean water supply and sewerage. Since the Black Death, medicine had ceased to be the prerogative of the Church, with the result that quacks and illiterate practitioners flourished. An Act of 1512 sought to regularize medical practice by requiring examination for proficiency, conducted by the bishop of the diocese and such experts as he might appoint; this led to the foundation of the College of Physicians in 1518. In these reforms Henry, himself a skilled amateur physician, played his part.

But from 1527 his character started to change, until the brilliant young man gave place to the morose and bitter tyrant. Part of this change was undoubtedly due to the worries of his divorce from Katherine, for the arguments lasted no less than six years. The first definite sign of imbalance is seen in 1531, when Henry permitted enactment of the new and frightful punishment of boiling to death. At least three people were executed by this means. Within a few months of Henry's death, the Act was repealed by the advisers of Edward VI. In 1533 came the first 'treason act' by which any person who cast a slander on the marriage with Anne Boleyn or who tried to prejudice the succession of its issue was guilty of treason.

Henry's reign of terror began in 1534 with an indiscriminate slaughter of Lollards, Lutherans, Anabaptists and Catholics. This was followed in 1535 by the barbarous execution of the prior of the Charterhouse and his monks, and the beheading of the saintly Thomas More and John Fisher. On 17 January 1536, Henry suffered a severe injury while jousting and lay unconscious for over two hours; he is said to have recovered by 4 February. This injury is the basis for the contention that Henry was essentially 'punch drunk'; but it occurred nine years after the first character change became manifest. By now Henry was definitely abnormal. His treatment of Anne Boleyn was savage. Head of the Church of England, he could easily have divorced her; he preferred to put her to death and also to divorce her by declaring her daughter a bastard. The suppression of the monasteries in 1538-40 was marked by the hanging of any abbot who dared to resist or delay his submission. The unnecessary vandalism, in which so much of the mediaeval art of England was wantonly destroyed, would surely never have been countenanced by the brilliant, learned young scholar who mounted the throne in 1509.

During these years of repression, Henry suffered from continual headaches and insomnia, from sore throats, and from the ulcer or fistula in his leg. In May 1538, at the age of forty-seven, he 'was sometime without speaking, black in the face and in great danger'. The French ambassador, Castillon, who reported this incident, associated the attack with closure of the fistula in the leg. For this reason it has been suggested that Henry suffered from a pulmonary embolism, blockage of the pulmonary artery by a blood clot from a varicose vein. The loss of speech is more in favour of an apoplectic fit.

In 1539 came the Statute of Six Articles, a piece of legislation against those who challenged Henry's position as 'Head of the Church in England' rendering a Protestant liable to be burned as a heretic and a Roman Catholic liable to be hanged as a traitor. Henry's vacillating policy as to the extent of religious reform was probably dictated by the changing opinions of his several wives and their 'parties' rather than by his own mind. There is no doubt that Henry's chagrin over the ugliness of Anne of Cleves, introduced to him by the reforming party, led directly to the downfall of Thomas Cromwell, endangered his friend and supporter Cranmer, and resulted in a renewed persecution of Protestants. The impression given is that Henry started out with the intention of reforming what was now his own Church and then took fright at the possible consequences to his soul on the Day of Judgement. There is here the suggestion of a split mind, one part endeavouring to present itself as a loyal son of Holy Mother Church, the other part intent on bending that Church to his own will.

Henry never lost his grip on affairs of state; in fact, after the fall and death of Wolsey in 1529, he tended towards an absolute rather than a constitutional monarchy. Only three years before his death, he led his army in person during the war with France and actively superintended the measures to combat an attempted invasion of England. Although prematurely aged, white-haired, monstrously obese, he never decayed into a physical and mental wreck. Nor did Henry die as Ivan died, terrified and delirious. The accounts of his death vary and the actual cause is obscure, but he died peacefully holding the hand of Archbishop Cranmer, the only friend who remained devoted to him to the last.

There is nothing indisputably diagnostic of syphilis in Henry's case history, but there is much that is suspicious: the headaches and sore throats, the pains in the joints, the ulcer in his leg which could have been a syphilitic inflammation of bone or its membrane, the 'fit' at forty-seven years, the suggestion of sterility, and, above all, the change in character which transformed his glorious youth into the cruelty of middle age.

A modern medical student is taught to look for the simple things before turning to 'the small print'. If faced with a fifteen-year-old boy suffering from a temperature, abdominal pain, and tenderness in the right flank, he should exclude acute appendicitis before considering a rarer condition. The story of Henry is exactly similar. His own history, the obstetric history of his wives, the suspicious death of Edward, the disabilities of Mary, even the short-sightedness of Elizabeth, all these are pointers. All of them can be separately explained by invoking a number of different ailments. But the evidence is cumulative. Syphilis was a common disease at the beginning of the sixteenth century, and the simple explanation is that Henry suffered from it.

Whatever the nature of Henry's disease (or combination of diseases), it exerted a profound effect upon the future of England. His failure to produce a healthy male line was the beginning of the end of the strong Tudor dynasty. There were no grandchildren, legitimate or illegitimate. The efficient rule of the Tudors gave way to the attempted absolutism of the weaker Stuarts that plunged the country into civil war.

After Henry's death in 1547, the nine-year-old Edward came to the throne under the guardianship of his mother's family, the Seymours. Under Seymour patronage, Edward became the champion of Protestants. Henry's despoliation of monastic property was completed even more ruthlessly. The bulk of monastic lands, treasure, and revenues was grabbed by greedy nobles. The reign of Edward is characterized by naked rapacity.

There was still considerable affection for the Old Faith. The fanatical iconoclasm of Edward's reign did not endear Protestantism to the ordinary Englishman. Had his successor and half-sister Mary behaved with moderation she might well have succeeded in restoring the Roman Catholic Church, perhaps not to its former power but lastingly as the official English religion. There is no doubt that Mary persisted in her persecutions despite warnings, especially by her Catholic husband Philip II of Spain. Had she quietly burned half a dozen rabid Protestants a year, she would have been honoured as a defender of the pure faith against heresy. But Mary, who was almost certainly mentally abnormal, would not listen to reason; she caused over 300 simple men and women to die at the stake in a little over three years, and she thereby ensured that the great majority of British people would regard Roman Catholicism as more evil than paganism. The settlement under

Elizabeth I came too late; religious toleration was unthinkable for over 200 years.

Mary's mental abnormality, whether caused wholly or in part by cerebral syphilis or whether the simple result of her traumatic childhood, so profoundly stirred religious thought in Britain that the effect is evident today. Indeed, it is still difficult to find the truth of many incidents in the sixteenth and seventeenth centuries, for the account given by a Protestant writer will materially differ from that of a Catholic. Those distant fires still smoulder on in Northern Ireland in the battles between Protestant and Roman Catholic. The Marian persecution also helped to crystallize the Englishman's thoughts on suffering. Britain and her cousin America have always honoured valour but, unlike some other countries, have never taken kindly to the idea that there is anything particularly noble in the voluntary bearing of pain. It is for this reason that the flagellant movement gained no adherents in England; it is for this reason that the merciful science of anaesthesia found its first practitioners in America and Britain. The agony of the sixteenth-century martyrs aroused not only anger and pity but also disgust. These tortures were borne voluntarily; the sufferer would have been spared by a simple recantation, in most cases involving nothing more than a reversion to doctrines accepted during earlier life. For the majority of Englishmen, the mediaeval ideal of a glorious martyrdom perished in the fires of sixteenth-century Smithfield.

The earliest known treatment of syphilis was by purgatives and the administration of semi-magic antidotes to poisoning. The first specific drug, guaiacum, remained a popular remedy until the end of the sixteenth century, although attacked by Paracelsus, one of the more revolutionary physicians. These treatments must have been quite ineffective. A much more efficient though dangerous drug was found in mercury.

Mercury, in the form of the ore cinnabar, had been used in the treatment of skin disease by the Arabian school of doctors and an ointment of metallic mercury was prescribed by Theo-

doric of Lucca in the thirteenth century. Theodoric advised
a six-day course and he noted that it caused profuse salivation,
a sign of mercury poisoning. This early use of mercury has
been adduced as evidence that syphilis is an ancient disease
in Europe, while the lack of any mention of mercury treatment (a form of treatment that is difficult to hide) has suggested to some historians that Henry cannot have suffered
from syphilis. Neither argument is particularly convincing.
Mercury seems to have been used for any form of severe skin
disease. In Henry's case, mercury would not have been used
unless there was manifest skin involvement.

The first recorded mercurial treatment of syphilis is by
Giorgio Sommariva of Verona in 1496; Sommariva was not a
doctor. A little later Jacopo Berengario da Carpi, who attended Benvenuto Cellini, became famous throughout Italy for
his successful treatments with mercury. The method soon
became known as 'salivation', because of the immense quantities of saliva it produced. Mercury medication by ointments,
oral administration or vapour baths remained popular for
three centuries; it was fairly effective, if persisted in, but
dangerous and extremely unpleasant. For this reason many
attempts were made to find other specifics, but the only one to
prove of lasting value was potassium iodide, introduced in
the 1840s, which proved effective in the later stages of the
disease. Much harm resulted from the activities of quacks who
claimed to possess secret remedies, and an Act of 1917 made
treatment of syphilis by unqualified persons a criminal
offence in Britain.

The full history of the infection was not clearly understood
until the twentieth century. In 1905 two Germans, F. R.
Schaudinn and P. E. Hoffmann, discovered the causative
organism, to which they gave the name *Spirochaeta pallida*,
since changed to *Treponema pallidum*. Hideyo Noguchi, a
Japanese, isolated this organism from the brains of patients
who suffered from general paralysis of the insane, and thus
proved the link, half suspected for a century, between the
early and late stages of syphilis. In 1906-7 the Wassermann

test was developed, which showed the presence of the disease even when latent.

Four years after the discovery of the causative organism came one of the greatest of all medical advances. Ever since Joseph Lister first used carbolic acid in the treatment of wounds (1865) chemists and doctors had been searching for 'the perfect antiseptic', one which would destroy bacteria without injuring the human tissues. A selective bactericide of this type might be safely injected into the bloodstream. Many workers thought the idea to be a visionary one, but Paul Ehrlich of Frankfurt was convinced of its practicability. He conducted a number of experiments with various compounds; in his six hundred and sixth trial he, or his Japanese assistant S. Hata, produced the first effective 'systemic antiseptic', a drug which was lethal to bacteria when injected yet not unduly harmful to the body. This, the famous '606', was an organic arsenic compound, arsphenamine, which became known as salvarsan. Ehrlich christened his drug 'the magic bullet' and hoped that it would be effective against many bacteria, but salvarsan soon proved useless except against the very important group of spirochaetes or treponemes. Nor was it so harmless to the human body as he had hoped, for it produced quite severe side-reactions. Over 300 experiments later, Ehrlich produced a safer drug, '914', neoarsphenamine or neosalvarsan. These organic arsenical preparations proved their worth in the 1914-18 war, when difficulty of control led to a rampant increase of syphilis among troops of all nations.

The next step in successful treatment is also associated with an important general advance in medicine. In 1928 Alexander Fleming, of St Mary's Hospital, London, isolated crude penicillin, the existence of which had been known for over fifty years. Fleming made little use of his discovery, which passed almost unnoticed; it was not until thirteen years later, in 1941, that the first clinical trial was made by Howard Florey and others at Oxford. Penicillin, the first of the antibiotic group of drugs, proved effective against a great many strains of bacteria and did not usually have toxic side-effects. In 1943 John Friend Mahoney of New York employed penicillin in the treatment of syphilis with very good results, and the more effective, shorter penicillin course soon replaced the arsenical compounds. Penicillin proved effective not only against syphilis, but also against gonorrhoea, the second of the major venereal infections.

Much more important than the treatment of individual cases is the control of venereal disease by social measures. This very difficult problem has been tackled especially well by the Swedes, and their legislation is the model upon which that of other countries is largely based. Legislation and better, more easily obtained treatment resulted in a steady and quite rapid fall in the number of infected people between 1917 and 1939. The special conditions of warfare tend to increase the risk of venereal infection. The fall in numbers was checked by the Second World War but was resumed in 1947 and continued until 1954. At that time venereal diseases seemed to have been brought under control throughout the Western world; the number of new cases decreased so rapidly that many clinics were closed. Since 1958 there has been a very marked deterioration. Partly as the result of carelessness and wider sexual freedom, and partly because penicillin-resistant strains of organisms have emerged, venereal disease is now an acute social problem.

4

General Napoleon
and General Typhus

Napoleon Bonaparte is a towering personality. But the Napoleonic adventure is as much a story of his armies as of the man himself. These armies, born of a nation devastated by revolution, emerged as the greatest fighting force since Rome, and subjugated the whole of Europe except Britain. The fate of Napoleon cannot be divorced from that of his soldiers, nor can the fate of his soldiers be divorced from that of Napoleon. The emperor's victorious career was ended by the destruction of his Grand Army, which had known almost unbroken success for nearly twenty years. It was brought to ruin in the late summer of 1812, partly through Napoleon's failure of judgement and partly by sickness. A number of diseases attacked the army during the campaign of 1812, but the primary and most destructive agent was an epidemic of the campaign disease known as continued fever or typhus.

Typhus fever is entirely different from typhoid fever. The latter is a water-borne disease caused by a bacillus. Typhus fever is a disease of dirt. The causative organism, *Rickettsia prowazeki*, belongs to a class of organisms which lies midway between the relatively large bacteria, easily seen under a high-powered microscope and which produce diseases such as typhoid, syphilis, and tuberculosis, and the viruses, which produce such diseases as smallpox and measles and which are so minute that they can be identified only with an electronic microscope. The organism is carried by lice. Lice are often found on animals or in the cracks and crannies of old buildings, but they can also infest unwashed bodies and the seams of dirty clothing.

This is why typhus acquired the name of gaol fever and, since fevers were supposed to be caused by bad smells, this is the reason why English judges customarily bear small nosegays of sweet-smelling flowers to this day. The disease originated in the filthy prisons and spread from the felon in the dock to the judge upon the bench. Three such 'assize epidemics' occurred in the sixteenth century. These epidemics were late incidents in the history of typhus. The origin of the disease remains obscure. One theory holds that it originated in the East as an infection of lice and rats but subsequently became an infection of lice and men. Cyprus and the Levant were probably the first focus of spread to Europe, the earliest known severe outbreak being in the Spanish armies of Ferdinand and Isabella during 1489-90.

Since typhus is a campaign and dirt disease, particularly liable to occur in conditions where a number of people are herded closely together, wearing the same clothes for prolonged periods, and lacking means of ensuring bodily cleanliness, it sometimes had profound effects upon the fortunes of war. A remarkable example is the relatively small and localized epidemic which destroyed a French army besieging Naples in July 1528, thus making a decisive contribution to the final submission of Pope Clement VII to Charles V of Spain. Typhus also forced the Imperial armies of Maximilian II to break off the campaign against the Turks in 1566. Soldiers carried typhus fever across Europe during the Thirty Years War of 1618-48 and it was during this period that the disease became firmly established.

Typhus remained endemic in the whole of Europe from the seventeenth to the late nineteenth century, but it was only in conditions of warfare, extreme poverty or famine that major outbreaks occurred. The United States was not infected until early in the nineteenth century; a great epidemic occurred at Philadelphia in 1837. But the history of typhus is complicated by the existence of more than one form of the disease. 'True' typhus fever, characterized by high fever, delirium, a crisis, and a blotchy rash, is very dangerous. Other less dangerous variants are Rocky Mountain Spotted Fever, Brill's Disease—a mild type which occurred among New York Jews and was described by Nathan Edwin Brill in 1898 —and the Trench Fever of the First World War. This last variant, which was very prevalent among German and Allied troops, apparently replaced 'true' typhus in the armies it infected, for 'true' typhus did not occur among them, though it wrought havoc among the Serbs and Russians. After the Russian revolution and the civil war which followed, famine and disease devastated almost the whole country. Approximately 20 million cases of true typhus occurred in European Russia alone between 1917 and 1921, with from $2\frac{1}{2}$ million to 3 million deaths.

The mode of transmission of typhus by the bite of the infected body louse was first described in 1911. H. da Roche Lima isolated the causative organism in 1916 and named it after an American, Howard Taylor Ricketts, and an Austrian, Stanislaus Joseph von Prowazek, both of whom died while investigating the disease. Since then improvements in hygiene and the use of DDT to kill lice have brought typhus under control, but mystery still surrounds this disease, for it seems that very special conditions are necessary before it will flourish in a virulent form, even when there is gross infesta-

84

tion with lice. Typhus seems to require concomitant malnutrition and sordid living conditions before it will produce a lethal epidemic. We must hope that we shall be able to institute and maintain a world-wide standard sufficiently high to make the reappearance of this terrible disease impossible.

The fall of Napoleon was not inevitable. Given time, patience, and a measure of luck, he could have extended his empire to the East, consolidated his administration, and forced the British into impotent isolation, impregnable upon the seas but probably helpless to intervene upon the Euro-Asian land mass. Ill-luck and impatience were primarily responsible for the defeat of Napoleon's army.

In the spring of 1812, Napoleon had reached the height of his power and his glory. His empire spread eastward to the Russian frontier and to Austria; on the north, west, and south it was bounded by the North Sea, the Atlantic and the Mediterranean. Two of his brothers wore crowns, Joseph as King of Spain and Jerome as King of Westphalia. One sister was Grand Duchess of Tuscany, another the Princess Borghese, a third, who had married his marshal Achille Murat, now sat beside her husband on the throne of Naples. Eugène, son of his first wife, Josephine de Beauharnais, acted as Viceroy of Italy. Napoleon himself, having divorced Josephine in 1809, had contracted a brilliant marriage with the great-niece of Marie Antoinette, the Archduchess Marie Louise, daughter of Francis, last Holy Roman Emperor and first Emperor of Austria. To this union had been born on 20 March 1811 his first legitimate child and heir, who had immediately been accorded the title of King of Rome.

All this family splendour and imperial prestige ended at the sea coasts. No means had been found to cross the narrow channel, only twenty miles wide—less than a day's land march —which separated the Empire of France from England. The British navy barred the way. Further, the insolent British had recently managed to establish a base in Portugal and, having entrenched themselves behind the strongly fortified lines of Torres Vedras, demonstrated the possibility of maintaining and supplying an army by sea. But England was still vulnerable by land. A large part of her trade and the bulk of her wealth derived from India, then administered by the Honourable East India Company. The French navy could not intercept and capture the great merchant ships of 'John Company', which bore the riches of India to Britain. Britain needed money to carry on the war. The taking of India itself would not only deny her that money, but would also immeasurably harm her prestige. The overland route would be long and hard, but the prize which lay at the end of the road would be worth almost any sacrifice to win.

Napoleon had already tried the southern route to India, across the Mediterranean, through Egypt and Arabia to the Indian Ocean. That adventure ended at Aboukir Bay in August 1798, when Horatio Nelson inflicted a heavy defeat upon the French navy, thus transforming the Mediterranean into a British lake. The French army, cut off in Palestine, was ravaged by bubonic plague and only succeeded in returning to Europe with great difficulty. Aboukir proved that seaborne invasion was too dangerous to be practical. The conquest of India and the East could only be attained with the help of Russia or after her defeat and submission.

On 25 June 1807, ten days after gaining a military victory over the Russians, Napoleon met Tsar Alexander I at Tilsit and concluded a treaty of everlasting friendship. Six months later Napoleon outlined his plan for a combined Franco-Russian invasion of India through Turkey and Persia. The moment was propitious. Napoleon had beaten every enemy by land and at that time the British had not yet secured a base in Portugal. He had sufficient forces at command; with supplies and military aid from Russia, the campaign might prove no worse than a long and difficult route march.

The abnormal psychological make-up engendered by absolutism is seldom conducive to easy negotiation. Given a cooperative France, Alexander had everything to gain by helping Napoleon and simultaneously extending his realms to the Dardanelles, the Balkans and the China Sea. Given a co-operative Russia, Napoleon could certainly have stabilized his European conquests, fed his peoples from the vast corn-lands of eastern Europe, tapped the wealth of India, fortified his coasts and contemptuously resigned the empty dominion of the seas to the British navy. The scheme held a fair chance of success and, if successful, must have resulted in an impregnable Franco-Russian domination of the whole of Europe and Asia. But the essential trust and co-operation were lacking. The potential victors fell out over the division of spoils before the spoils had been won. Alexander demanded Constantinople and the Dardanelles as the minimum payment for Russia's help. Napoleon, looking forward to the reconquest of the Mediterranean and the Straits of Gibraltar, refused to envisage a solid Russian entrenchment on his eastern flank. The all too short propitious moment was wasted in sterile argument. In May 1808 Napoleon found himself faced with a Spanish insurrection; in August a British expeditionary force defeated Marshal Jean Junot at Vimiera in Portugal and the opening shots of the Peninsular War had been fired. Napoleon, forced to acknowledge that he had for the present a full-scale war in Europe on his hands, transferred the bulk of his Grand Army to Spain. Meanwhile Russia became entangled in a war with the Ottoman Empire, which engaged her for the next four years. The projected Grand Alliance was tacitly abandoned.

The two emperors concluded their conference at Erfurt in Germany on 14 October 1808, in an outwardly amicable fashion. But one great problem remained unsolved. In 1807 Napoleon had created the Grand Duchy of Warsaw, which Alexander saw as a move to restore the Polish state and to detach it from Russia. At Erfurt Alexander assured Napoleon of his support in the event of war with Austria, but he did nothing to prevent that war, and did not move when it broke out in April 1809. His primary interest had now become the foiling of French ambitions in Poland. The question became acute in February 1810, when Alexander formally insisted that 'the kingdom of Poland shall never be restored'. Napoleon wrote in the margin of the despatch: 'Divinity alone can speak as Russia proposes.'

Another and more intimate cause of friction had arisen

between the two emperors. Napoleon's marriage was child-less, yet Josephine had borne children by her previous marriage with de Beauharnais. Napoleon suspected that he could not beget children, a suspicion that was widely shared in France. His doubts were resolved in 1807 when his mistress Eléonore Denuelle bore him a son, and this was followed by another illegitimate child from Maria Walewska. Napoleon now asked for Anna, the fifteen-year-old sister of Tsar Alexander, but came up against the powerful Dowager Empress of Russia, who not only hated the French alliance but had heard and believed the rumour of his impotence. Finally, in 1810, Napoleon abruptly ended these negotiations by making a formal offer to the Austrian ambassador for the hand of the Archduchess Marie Louise Hapsburg. The offer was immediately accepted.

This dramatic *volte-face* was a symptom rather than the cause of breach between Russia and France. Ever since Tilsit, Alexander had faced the hostility of his nobles, who derived a large part of their wealth from the sale of timber to maritime countries, especially Britain. Napoleon's Continental System of trade, reinforced by the British blockade of Europe, cut off that source of income. In December 1810 Alexander, who until now had acquiesced in the System, issued an imperial *ukase* imposing a high tariff on French goods and opening Russian ports to neutral shipping. As Britain controlled the seas, this was equivalent to permitting unrestricted trade with the principal enemy of France. Russia had opted out of the Continental System and out of the French alliance.

It now seems obvious that in 1810-11 Napoleon should have consolidated his empire by clearing his threatened western flank. The British, though strongly entrenched within their fortified lines, could not muster a force of more than 30,000 men. There can be little doubt that Napoleon, by throwing everything that he had against them, could have driven the British from Europe. But such a campaign would have been long, costly, and inglorious. A military dictator cannot be forced into dull, unprofitable warfare; if he is to survive he must repay his people's sacrifices with dramatic successes. To the east lay the possibility of a brilliant series of dashing battles, and, at the end, the gilded cupolas and barbaric splendours of Moscow. Beyond Moscow the road led to the gorgeous East. Napoleon was a narcissist and something of an exhibitionist—even the simple uniform that he habitually wore as Emperor was a point of contrast amidst the gold-bedizened and multicoloured uniforms of his staff officers. He commissioned the Italian artist Canova to sculpt a statue of his body, naked except for a fig leaf. He designed his own gem-laden coronation robes. In Egypt he considered conversion to the Muslim faith and donned the flowing garb of an Arab chief. Perhaps it was the jewelled turbans, the diamond aigrettes, the opportunity of wearing exotic ceremonial apparel which drew Napoleon towards India, as much as or even more than the chance of dealing a humiliating blow to England.

So Napoleon committed the fatal mistake of sacrificing reality for a dream. In January 1812 he denuded Spain of many seasoned troops to reinforce his eastern armies. Napoleon commonly spoke of his campaign as 'the Polish War'. France was to appear as the saviour of a Poland enslaved by Russia. But he proclaimed to his troops, 'the peace which we shall conclude ... will terminate the fatal influence which Russia for fifty years has exercised in Europe.' And he told his ambassador to Russia, Armand de Caulaincourt, 'I have come to finish once and for all with the colossus of the barbarian North.' Early in 1812, he privately revealed his true ambition to the Comte de Narbonne: 'Alexander [the Great] was as far as I am from Moscow when he marched to the Ganges.' Narbonne thought the idea to be half-way between Bedlam and the Pantheon.

From August 1811 onwards Napoleon made preparation on a vast scale for the invasion of Russia. In March 1812 he induced Prussia and Austria to sign agreements providing troops for his adventure. In April he made the obvious move of offering a peace treaty with Britain, but he met with no success. Tsar Alexander wisely secured his northern and southern flanks by ending his Turkish war and by inducing the Prince Royal of Sweden to bring his country over to the side of Russia in return for promised aid against Norway.

Napoleon's armies assembled in cantonments which stretched across Europe from northern Germany to Italy, and, in June 1812, started their concentration in east Germany. The force numbered 368,000 infantry, 80,000 cavalry, 1,100 guns and a reserve of 100,000 men. During the campaign, reinforcements brought the total of troops involved to well over 600,000. For the first time in his career Napoleon had an overwhelming numerical majority: the Russian armies numbered slightly less than a quarter of a million.

Legend has it that almost the whole of Napoleon's enormous array was destroyed in the retreat from Moscow. But the legend is wrong. A much larger number of men perished on the outward march through Poland and west Russia than on the retreat. Excluding the flanking forces, mainly German and Austrian, Napoleon's central or task army numbered about 265,000 men. Only 90,000 of these reached Moscow.

At first everything went well. The summer was unusually hot and dry; the men could march quickly over easy roads. In east Germany the slow-moving supply columns kept slightly ahead of the main force; food was abundant and close at hand and the health of the troops remained uniformly good. Military hospitals had been set up in Magdeburg, Erfurt, Posen, and Berlin but there was little demand for their services. On 24 June 1812, the army encamped on the west bank of the River Niemen, the boundary between Poland and Prussia. Here Napoleon passed his army in dazzling review. Then his troops marched down to the river and crossed over narrow pontoons erected by the bridge-building engineers. Four days later the army reached Vilna. Napoleon slept in the room vacated by Alexander a week earlier.

Poland was filthily dirty. The peasants were unwashed, with foul matted hair, lousy and flea-ridden. Their miserable hovels abounded with insects. An abnormally hot, dry summer had affected the wells; water was hard to come by and thick with organic matter. The enemy now lay in front and the supply trains had to move at the rear of the fighting forces. The rudimentary roads of Poland were either soft with loose dust or rutted from the spring rains, causing the wagons to lag behind so that food became scarce. The huge army—much too large for coherent command—lacked efficient discipline. Only the best units were accustomed to long, ordered marches; these columns moved in a compact military formation, but the greater part of the army dissolved into straggling, undisciplined bands. Despite stringent orders and harsh punishments, this multitude of stragglers were forced by hunger to pillage the cottages, livestock and fields of the peasants, their nominal allies. The Poles can hardly be blamed if they did not accept the French as their liberators from the Russian tyrant. The supplies, the auxiliary troops, the guerilla fighters, upon which Napoleon had counted, failed to materialize. Instead, the eternal pillaging by his half-starved armies aroused a sullen fury which was to recoil upon his soldiers during the retreat.

If the war of liberation had been already lost, so had the chance of an easy victory over Russia. Nearly 20,000 horses, twice the number that might be expected to fall in a single major battle, died from lack of water and forage on the road to Vilna. Hunger-weakness and polluted water produced the common campaign diseases of dysentery and enteric fevers. New hospitals were established at Danzig, Königsberg, and Thorn, but they were unable to cope with the mob of returning sick. Then, just after the crossing of the Niemen, there appeared a few cases of a new and terrible malady. Men developed a high temperature and a blotchy pink rash, and their faces assumed a dusky blue tinge; many of those affected died very quickly. Typhus fever held the army in a fatal grip.

Typhus had been endemic in Poland and Russia for many years. There is no evidence that the French armies encountered it before 1812, and they had certainly never suffered a major epidemic. Their medical and sanitary arrangements, brilliantly organized under the direction of the great military surgeon Baron D. J. Larrey, were the finest in the world but could not possibly cope with disease upon the scale which now resulted. Preventive measures proved useless when the cause of infection was unknown. Lack of water and insufficient changes of clothing made bodily cleanliness impossible. Fear of Russian attack and Polish reprisals caused the men to sleep close together in large groups. The lice of infested hovels crept everywhere, clung to the seams of clothing, to the hair, and bore with them the organisms of typhus. At the time of the battle of Ostrovna, in the third week of July, over 80,000 men had perished from sickness or were too ill for duty. Disease alone had robbed Napoleon's central force of nearly a fifth of its effective strength by the end of the first month; his army was about 150 miles from the frontier and Moscow was 300 miles away.

There had, of course, been wastage from battle casualties as well as from disease, though not upon the same scale. The Russians had no supreme commander or overall strategic plan, and their two armies, led by Barclay de Tolly and Prince Bagration, acted independently. Nevertheless, Barclay de Tolly just managed to elude Napoleon at Vilna, and Jerome Bonaparte and Marshal Davout failed to entrap Bagration on the right wing. Fierce battles were fought by Murat at Ostrovno and by Davout at Moghilev—the headquarters of Tsar Nicholas in the First World War—but still the Russians managed to disengage. Napoleon believed that the Russian forces would join to make a stand at Vitebsk, and this had been their original plan. On 27 July he established contact with de Tolly's army, but on the same day de Tolly learned that Bagration had determined on a retreat to Smolensk. During the night de Tolly succeeded in slipping away while Napoleon was still preparing for battle.

This successful withdrawal had the effect of frightening the more cautious of the French leaders. On 28 July Louis Berthier, Joachim Murat, and Eugène de Beauharnais sought a conference with Napoleon. They must have sensed that the failure of the Russians to stand and fight was drawing the French army into a most dangerous situation. They told Napoleon that the wastage of troops through sickness and by desertion from the less reliable units had reduced the effective fighting strength to little more than half and that the difficulty of provisioning even this depleted force in a hostile countryside was formidable. They implored Napoleon to halt the march. Having listened to their arguments, he agreed to announce the end of the campaign of 1812. But the urgent need of a spectacular victory caused him to change his mind. Two days later Napoleon reversed his decision and told the generals: 'The very danger pushes us on to Moscow. The die is cast. Victory will justify and save us.'

So the sick, half-starved army struggled on. Just over two weeks later, on 17 August, they came in sight of Smolensk and the River Dnieper. Here the two Russian armies had joined and it seemed that they would at last stand. Napoleon, determined to destroy his elusive enemy, did not hurry to press the attack home. He ordered a frontal bombardment of Smolensk, while sending Junot forward across the Dnieper to cut the Russian line of retreat to Moscow. Barclay de Tolly learned of his danger in time and, having fired the buildings of Smolensk, he hastily retreated. On 19 August Junot brought the Russians to battle at Valutino, ten miles northeast of Smolensk; the French suffered 6,000 casualties but failed to halt the Russian retreat.

Smolensk was the point of no return. Moscow lay 200 miles off. If the eastern dream was to be realized, Napoleon must go forward whatever the cost. A return now would be to acknowledge humiliating defeat. These were the alternatives facing Napoleon, but some historians believe that he had a third and more hopeful course: to stop at Smolensk and give his army time to recover.

Napoleon had acquired a considerable knowledge of, and fully understood, the importance of public health measures. He showed great interest in Edward Jenner's discovery of vaccination as a preventive of smallpox. He had had his own son vaccinated when eight weeks old and encouraged a campaign for the vaccination of children and army recruits. No one as yet appreciated the relationship between lice and typhus fever, but lousiness had been regarded as a shameful sign of dirty habits for centuries. Samuel Pepys cannot be accounted the most cleanly of men, but lousiness was unusual enough to be recorded in his diary on 23 January 1669: '... when all comes to all she [his wife] finds that I am lousy having found in my head and body above twenty lice little and great, which I wonder at, being more than I have had I believe these twenty years.' Pepys changed all his clothes and cut his hair short 'so shall be rid of them'.

This cure for lousiness was as well known to Napoleon and his medical officers as to Pepys. Smolensk had been partially destroyed by fire but shelter could have been improvised by the engineers. The supply line to Germany and France was open and could have been kept open. A winter of rest, good rations, ample water supplies, medical care and sanitary control would have restored the broken army, allowed time for the reinforcement of men and commissariat, and might have enabled Napoleon to consolidate his position in Poland in order to launch an overwhelming attack on Russia in the summer of 1813. J. R. L. de Kerckhove, one of Napoleon's surgeons, later wrote that if Napoleon had been content to play this waiting game, his campaign might have been successful and his domination of central and eastern Europe permanently established.

Apart from Napoleon's character, there are still two reasons why this sensible third course did not appeal to him. First his armies had encountered difficulties in the Peninsular War. In July Wellington had gained a resounding victory over General Auguste Marmont at Salamanca, and in August had entered Madrid. Napoleon could not foresee that these successes would end, if only temporarily, in Wellington's costly and dispiriting winter retreat to Ciudad Rodrigo. The second reason is that Napoleon had convinced himself that the fall of Moscow must force Alexander to capitulate. He decided to make Smolensk an advanced base for the concentration of reserve troops and supplies and to set up similar bases at Minsk and Vilna. The road back was secure and Napoleon free to push on as quickly as possible to Moscow. He resumed the march on 25 August. But nearly half of his central columns had fallen by the way and his striking force now consisted of only 160,000 men. Typhus raged throughout the army. Less than a fortnight later, on 5 September, only 130,000 men remained.

Meanwhile, on 30 August, Alexander had appointed the veteran Prince Michael Kutusov commander-in-chief of the Russian armies. Kutusov had led the Russian division at Austerlitz in 1805, where he acquired a healthy respect for Napoleon as an opponent and gained some knowledge of his strategy. He continued to give ground, slowly withdrawing as the French advanced. On 5 September, the Russians came to the banks of the Moscow River, fifty miles to the south-east of the city. Kutusov would have preferred to continue a planned retreat, relying upon the wide, barren spaces of Russia and the imminent bitter cold of winter to destroy the French, but at least a token defence of the capital was demanded. Karl von Clausewitz, the great Prussian strategist and military historian, wrote:

Kutusov, it is certain, would not have fought at Borodino where he obviously did not expect to win. But the voice of the Court, of the Army, of all Russia, forced his hand.

Kutusov did not risk the whole of his command. The Russian forces at Borodino numbered 120,000 men, but 10,000 of these were raw, hastily trained militia. Opposing them were 130,000 seasoned French troops with 600 guns; the Russian artillery was slightly superior in number and weight. Kutusov entrenched his men on a slope above the Moscow River, centring them upon the village of Borodino, and prepared redoubts for his cannon. There, for two days, the army awaited battle.

The engagement which followed bore some resemblance to Waterloo, probably for the same reasons. Napoleon was a sick man at Waterloo, unable to give his whole attention to the battle. The same is true of Borodino. He was in great pain from an acute attack of cystitis, inflammation of the bladder, and had difficulty in passing water. He also suffered from a heavy, feverish cold. His illness probably accounts for the delay of two days in attacking the Russian position, but the question arises: how far was Napoleon in charge of the battle and to what extent, if any, did his sickness affect the issue? He disregarded Davout's advice to attempt an encircling movement by turning the Russian left wing, which would seem a sensible method of destroying an entrenched army. The excuse has been made that Napoleon had already experienced the Russians' agility in disengaging themselves when threatened on the flank. Whatever the reason, the French mounted a massive cavalry attack upon the well-defended Russian centre, the same tactics which Marshal Michel Ney employed against the unbroken British line at Waterloo.

Battle was joined at dawn on 7 September. The French cavalry charged repeatedly, but the Russians succeeded in re-forming; not until evening were they at last driven from their entrenched position. At the height of the battle, when it seemed that a spectacular Russian defeat was within reach, Davout urged Napoleon to throw in the Imperial Guard. He refused. Many of his generals questioned this decision but Napoleon countered their criticism with the words: 'If I throw in the Guard, with what shall I fight tomorrow?' Whether through his foresight or by chance, the decision to withhold his best troops prevented a complete disaster two months later.

Both sides suffered heavy casualties, the French losing some 30,000 men and the Russians 50,000. Obviously the French loss was more serious, since they were operating in hostile territory. But at least it was victory of a kind, though in the long term meaningless. The Russians retired, retained freedom to manoeuvre, and had the certainty of receiving ample supplies and reinforcements. Kutusov clearly appreciated the situation. He had fought his token battle for Moscow and withdrawn in good order. Disease, cold, and hunger would effectively do his work for him. On 13 September he held a council of war. 'The salvation of Russia is in her army,' he argued. 'Is it better to risk the loss of the army and of Moscow by accepting battle, or to give up Moscow without a battle?' His argument was unanswerable and the army retreated through the city in a south-easterly direction towards the town of Ryazan.

The French therefore marched unopposed to Moscow. But typhus marched with them. Their army of just under 100,000 men suffered nearly 10,000 casualties by sickness in the week 7-14 September. Of over 300,000 who had formed and re-inforced Napoleon's central force, only 90,000 reached Moscow. Seven out of every ten had fallen by the way. On 14 September the tattered remnant of the army saw the gilded and multicoloured domes shining before them. All the church bells were ringing; Napoleon expected to be met by a deputation of leading citizens, offering him the keys of the city. The gates remained shut. That primitive but effective siege engine, the battering-ram which had been dragged across the length of Poland, was brought forward. The gates were battered down and the army entered, to find empty streets and silent houses. Within a few hours, fires broke out in several districts.

The true story of these fires will probably never be known. The population of Moscow numbered about 300,000. For some days the governor, Count Rostopchin, had been organizing the evacuation of the city; by the time of Napoleon's entry, rather less than 50,000 remained. Immense quantities of stores and personal possessions were also removed. In the last phase of evacuation, Rostopchin released prisoners from the city gaols. Legend has it that he released them on condition that they harass the French by pillaging and arson. Rostopchin's action in sending all fire engines out of the city suggests that the fires were deliberate rather than that they were caused by drunken citizens or French soldiers.

Napoleon, overjoyed that Moscow had been won, clung to his opinion that Alexander must now sue for peace. His judgement was at fault. Alexander could not submit; he had been warned by his sister on 19 September that the capture of Moscow had stiffened national feeling against the French to such an extent that peace negotiations might endanger his life. De Caulaincourt tried to convince Napoleon that Alexander neither would nor could accept defeat. He refused to act as intermediary; on 4 October Napoleon sent General Lauriston on a peace mission to St Petersburg.

Kutusov learned of Lauriston's embassy and ordered his Cossack patrols to fraternize with the French outposts, thereby lulling Napoleon into a false sense of security and providing a rational basis for his peace fantasy. Kutusov was playing for time. Nearly three-quarters of Moscow had been destroyed by fire. Typhus spread unchecked among the French, the sick finding such shelter as they could among the burnt-out ruins or in improvised shelters on the outskirts. Army morale fell to a low ebb; the soldiers, disappointed of the ample supplies which they had been promised, spent their time plundering and drinking the stocks of alcohol that remained in the city cellars.

The hot, dry summer passed into an abnormally warm autumn. De Caulaincourt, the one man in Napoleon's entourage who had experience of a Russian winter, warned Napoleon that his position in the ruined, wasted city must be untenable once the cold weather set in. Napoleon, misled by the unusually mild season, replied that de Caulaincourt was exaggerating; a Russian winter could be no worse than winter at Fontainebleau. Thus his futile peace parleys combined with a warm autumn to lead Napoleon into the final mistake of this disastrous campaign. The remnant of his army could only be saved by adopting one of two courses: either he must be content with an empty victory and return to Smolensk, or he might try to push north by forced marches in order to join up with his Prussian allies on the road to St Petersburg. A bold stroke against the capital would possibly have brought Russia to her knees.

The French had lost touch with the main body of the enemy. They thought that the Russians had retreated east; in fact, they rapidly marched in a half-circle south and west to cut Napoleon off from their main centres of supply and arms manufacture at Kaluga and Tula. Kutusov struck on

18 October, making a surprise attack upon Murat's force at the town of Tarutino, south of Moscow, forcing them to withdraw and inflicting 4,000 casualties. This comparatively small battle warned Napoleon that his peace bid had failed and that he was now in danger of encirclement. On 19 October his army began the retreat from Moscow.

Fifteen thousand reinforcements joined the French army during their month's stay in the city, but nearly 10,000 men succumbed to disease and wounds. The army which left Moscow on 19 October amounted to just over 95,000 dirty, half-starved, unhealthy men. They were encumbered with their sick and wounded, 600 cannon, and an immense mass of loot which included the enormous and quite useless gilded copper cross from the cupola of the tower called Ivan Veliki. Napoleon turned south in order to avoid the devastated direct road to Smolensk, intending to march back through Kaluga. On 24 October he encountered the Russians at Malojaroslavetz. A heavy day's fighting ended indecisively. Napoleon, having suffered 5,000 casualties, declined to press the attack next day; Kutusov also lost the opportunity of inflicting a decisive defeat.

The way south was barred; Napoleon had no option but to turn north and east, rejoining the Smolensk road at Borodino. The cold was now becoming intense and snow started to fall heavily on 5 November. Swiftly riding bands of Cossacks, aided by guerillas, rendered foraging almost impossible. No preparations had been made for a winter campaign. De Caulaincourt managed to obtain ice-shoes for the horses of Napoleon's suite, but not a single cavalry or artillery horse was properly shod. This, and not the cold, is the reason for Napoleon's despatch of 7 November, 'the cavalry is on foot'.

The army pressed on to the promised food and shelter of Smolensk. Napoleon arrived with the vanguard on 8 November, to find his reserves, under Claude Victor, wasted by typhus fever, and the hospitals already crowded with sick. Discipline had broken down to such an extent that rations could no longer be fairly distributed. The greatest blow of all was the almost complete lack of food, for the reserves and communication troops had consumed most of the supplies stored against the army's return. Finding no hope in Smolensk, Napoleon evacuated the city on 13 November, leaving over 20,000 sick in the makeshift hospitals and ruined houses. Next day he found the road at Krasnoi barred by Kutusov.

The Russians expected that the depleted French army would avoid battle, but Napoleon, in order to allow his straggling forces time to concentrate, hurled in the Imperial Guard. These valiant troops, preserved so carefully at Borodino, now prevented entire and humiliating military defeat. Kutusov, driven back by their fury, could not reform to attack. Leaving Ney to fight a magnificent rearguard action, Napoleon pushed on to his next supply base at Minsk. On 22 November he received the appalling news that Minsk had fallen to the enemy.

Two days later he learned that the Russians had destroyed his bridgehead over the River Beresina. The pontoon bridges had already been abandoned for lack of transport. The position seemed hopeless, for the flanking armies had been heavily defeated by Prince Wittgenstein in the north and by Admiral Tchitchagov in the south. The Russian pincers were closing in on either side and Kutusov's army blocked the way to the west. The situation was saved by a feigned crossing to the south of Studianka, which served to mislead Tchitchagov, while the brilliant engineer General Jean Baptiste Eblé improvised two bridges to the north. Despite the heroism of the rearguard, only 50,000 men were able to continue the retreat.

The army now began to degenerate into an undisciplined rabble. On 29 November Napoleon wrote:

Food, food, food—without it there are no horrors that this undisciplined mass will not commit at Vilna. Perhaps the army will not rally before the Niemen. There must be no foreign agents in Vilna; the army is not a good sight today.

Fifteen thousand men died on the road between the Beresina and Vilna. But there was worse in store.

The starving vanguard reached Vilna on 8 December, having marched through thickly falling snow driven by a bitter north-east wind. Only 20,000 sick and disheartened men comprised the effective force; the rest were stragglers, stumbling along as best they could, harried by Cossack patrols, starving and frozen. Of Ney's Third Corps, only twenty men remained. The town offered no relief. Already starving, it was crowded with sick, and typhus had spread throughout the surrounding countryside. Men suffering from typhus fever, dysentery, and pneumonia lay on rotten straw soaked with their own excrement, without medical attention or means of warmth, so hungry that they gnawed leather or even human flesh. By the end of December over 25,000 sick and frost-bitten men had struggled into the town; less than 3,000 of these were alive in June 1813.

On 5 November, Napoleon had received news from Paris of his rumoured death and of a conspiracy, led by General Claude François de Malet, to seize power. On 6 December, while at Smorgoni to the west of Vilna, he decided upon a hasty return to France before the full extent of the disaster could be realized. He drafted a bulletin for despatch to Paris in the usual manner; this gave a frank account of the horrors of the retreat but did not mention the complete breakdown of supply arrangements; blame was laid entirely upon the weather. Napoleon then set out, first by chaise, then on horse-back. After a furious ride across the whole of Germany and eastern France, he arrived at the Tuileries in Paris on the night of 18 December, anticipating his catastrophic bulletin by two days. He handled a dangerous, indeed desperate, situation with supreme skill, from the understatement of his report to the Senate on 20 December 1812: 'My army has had some losses, but this was due to the premature rigour of the season', to his successful mobilization of 470,000 new troops by the autumn of 1813. This, perhaps the most astonishing episode in Napoleon's astonishing career, bears witness to his tenacity and speed of action when faced with a threat to his power.

He could save himself but he could not save his army. Murat, left in command, proved a broken reed. He refused to make a stand at Vilna and, on 10 December, abandoned the last guns, the remaining baggage and the treasury to the Russians. On 12 December Berthier reported to Napoleon that the army no longer existed; even the Imperial Guard, now reduced to less than 500 men, had lost all semblance of a military formation. Ney, still fighting a stubborn rearguard action, crossed the Niemen on 14 December. When the last stragglers had shuffled over to the German bank, there remained less than 40,000 men of the brilliant Grand Army which Napoleon had reviewed on 24 June. It is said that only 1,000 of those who returned were ever again fit for duty. So ended Napoleon's dream fantasy, the conquest of Russia and of India. There were, of course, other causes of defeat besides typhus fever: cold, hunger, the Russians—and Napoleon Bonaparte himself.

Napoleon was born by a precipitate labour on 15 August 1769. Here is a picture of him in 1795, at the age of twenty-six: a small man, only five feet six inches tall, with a square face, a strangely sallow complexion, a well-formed nose, grey eyes, dark brown hair. His most striking physical characteristic at this age was his excessive thinness; although well-muscled and fairly powerful, he seemed a runt of a man. He had a lively, rather impressive expression when his interest was aroused, but at other times he often looked so miserable that people thought he must be in actual pain. In early life he took little care of his person: his long, ill-powdered hair hung over his coat collar; his clothes and boots were shabby, and his hands dirty. He had always been a bookish youth, intelligent and ready to learn, an excellent mathematician. In adolescence he had shown remarkably little interest in sex.

Napoleon's swift and dazzling rise to supreme power resulted from a combination of brilliant imagination, unusual intelligence tempered by downright common sense, and an acute perception of the correct moment for any particular course of action. His magnificent brain was as if divided into separate compartments which could be opened or closed whenever he wished. Thus, he dictated orders and plans to a number of secretaries, turning from one subject to another as he walked between their desks. His notorious anger was a calculated weapon to inspire fear, and was entirely under control. He lived for power and knew that power depends largely upon fear. 'Abroad and at home I reign only through the fear I inspire.' Later in his career, he was to imagine himself as his own ideal of a gloomy, cold-blooded, inaccessible tyrant, but he never achieved that ideal: although formidable, he remained fascinating. Talkative, gregarious, possessed of great charm which, like his anger, could be switched on or off at a moment's notice, he aroused a genuine love and devotion among those who came in contact with him. Even his enemies were impressed: the ship's company of the *Bellerophon* which took him to Saint Helena agreed that 'if the people of England knew him as well as we do, they would not hurt a hair of his head'. His veterans worshipped him, for his fantastic memory enabled him to call any one of them by name—and it was the duty of his aide-de-camp to prompt that memory should it fail.

Napoleon achieved his success by a phenomenal capacity for hard work. Pressure of work caused him to neglect his natural body requirements. He slept for only three hours each night and developed the ability, not uncommon among hard-pressed administrators, of falling deeply asleep for very short periods at intervals during the day. That master of gastronomy, Anthelme Brillat-Savarin, dismissed Napoleon as 'an undiscerning eater'. He bolted his food, often taking only twelve minutes over dinner, and ate when business permitted rather than at set hours. Despite this unhealthy regimen, Napoleon seems to have been remarkably fit during his earlier years in power.

He had, of course, certain disabilities which became more troublesome as he aged. The story of infertility, half suspected by himself, came to a happy end with the birth of his bastard sons. The rumour of epilepsy may have a firmer foundation. As a lad at Brienne he fell unconscious to the ground, but this was probably nothing more than a faint. During the near-disaster of Brumaire in November 1799, when he was physically attacked by infuriated members of the Five Hundred, he was dragged to safety in an almost unconscious state; this, again, was probably a mere 'faint' brought on by a quite unexpected crisis. But three attacks, which bear some resemblance to epileptic fits, are recorded as occurring between January 1803 and September 1805.

The suggestion has also been made that Napoleon suffered from syphilis; the story is based on some urinary trouble during the Consulate of 1802-4. Napoleon himself wrote that the opinion of his doctor, Alexis Boyer, caused him to 'conceive strange suspicions of Josephine, for I was quite sure of myself'. But his urinary symptoms (already noticed at the battle of Borodino) are more suggestive of small stones, 'gravel', in the bladder; there is little here to support a diagnosis of syphilis.

The most serious of Napoleon's early illnesses to be diagnosed with any certainty is migraine, the distressingly painful 'sick headache' which is all too common among highly-strung people who work at high pressure. The first report of migraine comes towards the end of the Italian campaign of 1796 and he suffered from attacks at moments of stress throughout his life. Another symptom of Napoleon's highly-strung temperament is his itching skin. This must have been a dermatitis of nervous origin but may have been induced by the true 'itch' or scabies which he contracted at Toulon in December 1793.

Two other disabilities, neither of them serious in itself, exerted a profound effect upon Napoleon's later career. Napoleon was certainly a man of 'irregular habits'. These resulted in obstinate constipation; the straining at stool, induced by constipation, rendered him liable to attacks of prolapsed haemorrhoids, or piles. The first mention of this common but painful ailment is in 1797 when he was twenty-eight years old. Five years later, in 1802, irregular eating habits produced another painful condition, equally common among those who live at high pressure and without due care. Fauvelet de Bourrienne, Napoleon's secretary, recorded that about the beginning of the year 1802 Napoleon began to suffer from pain in his right side. He would quite often lean against the right arm of his chair, unbutton his waistcoat, and exclaim, 'Oh what a pain I feel.' This may have been gall stone colic or even simple indigestion, but the later history is more typical of that bane of the harassed financier, a peptic ulcer.

In 1805 Napoleon, crowned emperor on 2 December 1804, was thirty-six years of age. From now on he started to deteriorate, both physically and mentally. This fairly rapid change was noticed by all those in contact with him. He began to fill out, to develop a paunch. His thin face became rounded and his neck thickened. The long straggling hair receded from his forehead, grew sparser and finer in texture. His skin was softer and smoother; his hands, once long and 'beautiful' (although dirty) became covered with fatty tissue and so gave the appearance of being small and pudgy. The lean, haggard Corsican Ogre of the James Gillray caricatures changed into the better-known stocky little Napoleon of school history-book pictures.

This physical change was accompanied by a marked alteration in temperament and mentality. Basically he lost self-discipline. From 1806 onwards his ministers were little better than yes-men. Denis Decrès, Minister of Marine, declared: 'The Emperor is mad and will destroy us all.' In 1807 Prince Metternich observed that 'there has recently been a total change in the methods of Napoleon; he seems to think that he has reached a point where moderation is a useless obstacle'. His temper was no longer under control; although his rages were less frequent, he was no longer capable of turning them on and off at will. He lost the common sense which had nearly always guided his actions; his rule not only became more absolute, but he allowed his fantasies to take charge of his plans. Hand-in-hand with lust for power and dream-fantasies there went an unwonted impatience. But the body refused to obey the dictates of the mind. His magnificent vitality slackened and he lost the capacity for prolonged constructive work. By the age of forty, Napoleon had changed into a lethargic and hesitant man.

What was the reason for this dramatic change? Many

theories have been advanced but not one wholly explains the facts. His obesity and lethargy suggest a physical rather than a mental cause; for this reason many medical historians believe that he suffered from a disorder of the thyroid gland. Thyroid deficiency, myxoedema, might produce a clinical picture of this nature, but the depicted features of Napoleon do not favour the diagnosis. Fröhlich's Syndrome, a deficient secretion of the pituitary gland at the base of the brain, has been suggested. But it is unlikely that a person suffering from this disease would be capable of siring children. Moreover, neither of these theories takes into account the three 'fits' or epileptiform convulsions of 1803-5. These are unlikely to have been symptoms of true epilepsy for there is no story of similar incidents in later life. The diagnosis of a low grade neurosyphilis cannot be summarily dismissed, but it is equally, if not more, possible that the fits were associated with his known migraine. Some patients who suffer from severe migraine have occasional epileptiform fits. Ordinary migraine can occasionally develop into the condition now called 'complicated migraine', in which fits or even paralyses and disturbances of speech can occur. These severe symptoms almost certainly result from spasm of the cerebral arteries; such spasm could easily lead to minor brain damage. If this were the case, Napoleon's lethargy would be the result of minor brain damage from complicated migraine and his obesity would, in turn, result from his lethargy. The damage must have been comparatively minor, for it is apparent that Napoleon could react violently and swiftly when faced with a direct challenge to his power, nor is there any evidence that he developed any of the grosser manifestations of severe brain damage. Whatever the cause may have been, and it is unwise to be dogmatic here, the new Napoleon lacked the quickness and decision of the old. Nevertheless, between December 1812 and July 1813 he gathered a force of 470,000 men. His army was superior in numbers to that of the Allies, but consisted of poor quality, raw recruits, a type always more susceptible to campaign diseases than seasoned veterans. The retreating French and the pursuing Russians had scattered typhus fever throughout the length and breadth of Germany; by the autumn of 1813 all central and eastern Europe was in the grip of a severe epidemic. Thousands of French soldiers succumbed until, by late autumn, less than half the army remained.

Nevertheless, the French scored victories at Lützen and Bautzen and, for a time, seemed on the point of inflicting decisive defeat upon the Allies at Dresden. After two days of bitter fighting, during which time Napoleon directed the battle in person, the Allied armies were forced to retreat, leaving the French poised for an annihilating stroke on the next day. But now one of Napoleon's comparatively minor disabilities attacked him and helped to change the course of history. On that evening of the second day of Dresden, Napoleon was exhausted, soaked to the skin, famished with hunger. He ate ravenously and during the night of August 27-8 pain and vomiting became so severe that he was forced to return to the rear, leaving Marshal Mortier, Marshal Laurent de St Cyr and General Dominique Vandamme to conduct the next day's battle. The defeat of Vandamme prevented a rout of the Allies.

Two months later, on 17 October, a similar attack of abdominal pain and vomiting prostrated Napoleon during the decisive battle of Leipzig, but in this case his illness probably did not affect the issue. The French were driven back across the Rhine; Wellington was fighting his way up from the Pyrenees; Prussians under Gebhard, Prince Blücher, Austrians under Prince Schwarzenberg, Russians under Tsar Alexander were pouring along the roads to Paris: the days of the Napoleonic Empire were numbered. At this critical, hopeless time something of Napoleon's old magic returned. Wellington said of the 1814 campaign that 'the study of it has given me a greater idea of his genius than any other'. 'But,' added Wellington, 'he wanted patience.' On 6 April 1814, the Marshals insisted upon unconditional abdication; on 11 April Napoleon made a declaration renouncing the thrones of France and Italy.

There followed the attempted suicide, probably by means

of strychnine, on the night of 12 April, the terrible journey through southern France when the fallen Emperor narrowly escaped lynching at Avignon and saw himself hanged in effigy at Orgon, and the exile as monarch of Elba. Here he seems to have been reasonably happy, administering his tiny kingdom, exercising his toy army, probably supported by his plans and his hopes. Then came the dramatic, almost insanely adventurous return to France. On 1 March 1815, Napoleon landed at Antibes and started upon his triumphant progress through Mouans-Sartoux, Grasse, Digne, Grenoble and Lyons back to Paris.

The ill-health which had now dogged him for ten years almost brought the venture to an end before it had really started. The returning hero rode triumphantly on horseback at the head of an impressive cavalcade from Antibes to Grasse. Here the haemorrhoids, which had troubled him on and off since 1797, became excruciatingly painful. Even to walk was agonizing, to ride a horse unthinkable. He commanded a carriage to be brought forward and for a time found some comfort, but the rough road and the jolting of the heavy wheels made relief only temporary. A sick and deposed monarch lolling up on cushions is very different from a returning conqueror prancing upon his war-horse. But the attack passed fairly quickly and, after two days, Napoleon found himself able to continue the march; had the illness been more prolonged, his triumphant progress might well have ended at Grasse.

These same troublesome piles, together with Napoleon's somnolence and lethargy, largely account for what the French still call 'the enigma of Waterloo'. Of all the armies which Napoleon recruited, that which fought at Waterloo was the one most needing coherent and inspiring command. They were 'a scratch lot', unaccustomed to their leaders, hastily enrolled during the Hundred Days. But the troops cannot be blamed for the disaster of Waterloo. Napoleon lost the battle of 18 June by losing his opportunity on 17 June. On the evening of 16 June, the strategic position looked most favourable for the French; this fact, considering the poor quality of his troops, itself bears testimony to Napoleon's skill as a commander.

Napoleon, commanding some 124,000 men, faced a Prussian army of 120,000 under Prince Blücher and a mixed British-Dutch-German-Belgian force of 100,000 under the Duke of Wellington. Napoleon's admirable plan was to operate with two wings and a large reserve. Headquarters having been set up at Charleroi, one wing under Marshal Ney was ordered to hold Wellington on the Brussels road, while the other wing, under General Emmanuel Grouchy, engaged the Prussians, still some ten miles to the east of the nearest point where they could make contact with their British allies and so face Napoleon with an overwhelming numerical superiority. Ney duly attacked the British at Quatre Bras; Grouchy and Napoleon broke and partially routed the Prussians at Ligny. Neither battle was decisive, but the possibilities for the following day were immense. Napoleon with the reserve could either complete the rout of the Prussians on the right, or could easily swing to the left and smash Wellington. But, as the military historian Becke has written, 'it was in these twelve hours from 9 p.m. on the 16th to 9 a.m. on the 17th that the campaign was lost'.

Napoleon had been in the saddle for the whole day of 16 June. This obese, prematurely-aged man of forty-six was completely worn out. Worse still, his piles had once more become agonizingly painful. Throughout the night of 16-17 June he remained sleepless, in pain. In the morning he did not leave his bed until eight. Not until 11 a.m. did he order Grouchy to pursue the Prussians. By now contact had been lost; Napoleon made the fatal mistake of ordering pursuit to the *east*, whereas Blücher had retired to the *north*. At the same time he ordered the Guard to move up in support at Quatre Bras. Wellington, having learned of Blücher's retreat to the north, moved the British force back up the Brussels road to parallel the Prussians and to establish a defensive position on the high ground before the village of Waterloo. For some hours the British were entangled in the narrow streets and single bridge of Genappe, an easy target for Ney's army.

Meanwhile Grouchy, feeling his way east and south, was every moment increasing his distance from the point of battle.

On 17 June the sun rises at about 3.45 a.m. G.M.T. Over four hours of daylight were wasted before Napoleon awoke from his uneasy sleep, over seven hours before he was in a fit condition to assume control of strategy. It is certain that he had the opportunity of inflicting decisive defeat; it is equally certain that he lost the chance. The young Napoleon would never have missed the opportunity offered: he would have risen triumphantly to the occasion, exhaustion or no exhaustion, pain or no pain; but the lethargic, impatient, pain-ridden Napoleon of June 1815 was no longer capable of the supreme effort required. To the medical historian, Saturday 17 June is the fatal day; the Sunday of Waterloo, with Napoleon still unable to exercise full control of the battle, comes as something of an anticlimax. Yet, for all his ill-health and the mistakes made by Ney, Napoleon very nearly defeated Wellington at Waterloo; if we accept the victor's own appreciation: 'It was the most desperate business I ever was in: I never took so much trouble about any battle, and never was so near being beat,' then Napoleon's ill-health may have provided the necessary weight to tilt the balance.

Six years later Napoleon died at St Helena, on 5 May 1821. Those six years were a time of hopeless frustration, of petty quarrelling, of sulky seclusion. Undoubtedly the governor, Sir Hudson Lowe, lacked the tact and the intelligence to handle so difficult a prisoner as Napoleon, but the legend of the 'Martyrdom of St Helena' has no basis of fact. Politically it was necessary for the British to present the island as something in the nature of a health-resort; politically it was necessary for Napoleon's sympathizers to present it as being more akin to Devil's Island. Even Pope Pius VII, whom Napoleon had arrested and exiled, made a plea for his release on the grounds 'that the craggy island of St Helena is mortally injurious to health, and that the poor exile is dying by inches'.

A form of liver disease, an acute infective hepatitis, was endemic on St Helena. Napoleon may have fallen sick of it;

but, if so, he quickly recovered. His terminal illness lasted for six months. Much has been written about it and many theories have been advanced. In fact, the history is quite clear. During his last days he suffered from 'tarry stools' and 'coffee-grounds vomit', both of which appearances are caused by digested or semi-digested blood. General Henri-Gratien Bertrand wrote of hiccups, vomiting, and the same tarry stools. The treatment given to him does not seem to have been very sensible: one of the last drugs administered was a large dose of calomel, which can have done not the slightest good and may have actually hastened death. The post-mortem reports vary as to the condition of Napoleon's liver, but all mention a large 'scirrhous growth' of the stomach. This, taken together with the history of tarry stools, coffee-grounds vomit and hiccups make the diagnosis of the cause of death quite certain. Napoleon died from a cancer of the stomach, which had pierced the wall, leaving an aperture sufficiently large to admit a finger. The cancer had eroded a blood vessel; death was due to exhaustion from haemorrhage and peritonitis, resulting from perforation of the stomach by the malignant growth. His end was a merciful one, for he might have lingered on to die from sheer starvation.

Although the cause of death is plain, allegations of poisoning were made. Napoleon, in his will, ordered that his head be shaved and locks of hair distributed to various followers. In 1960 it was reported that traces of arsenic had been shown to be present in samples of his hair. The truth will probably never be known, but poisoning by arsenic cannot possibly have been the immediate cause of death. Arsenic, however, is known to be one of the substances which may produce cancer and, if administered or taken inadvertently for any length of time, might have been the causative agent. It is conceivable but unlikely.

Napoleon died over five years after Waterloo and Waterloo was lost three years after the campaign of Moscow. But his disastrous fall began and became inevitable when his own health and judgement started to fail. His Grand Army was destroyed by his own impatience and by the ill-luck of encountering typhus fever, and his empire never recovered from the destruction of that army. On 29 November 1812, during the battle of the Beresina, Marshal Ney wrote to his wife: 'General Famine and General Winter, rather than the Russian bullets, have conquered the Grand Army.' This is the accepted opinion but, to make the picture complete, we should add the names of General Typhus and General Napoleon.

5
The Impact of
Infectious Diseases

So far we have considered diseases which seem to have originated in fairly primitive communities and to have exercised a devastating effect when carried to more civilized peoples. We turn now to those diseases which have developed in the more civilized countries, have become tamed by acquired resistance or by preventive treatment, yet have proved themselves lethal when accidentally transmitted to less highly developed peoples by the explorer, the missionary or the trader.

The mechanism is exactly the same whether the disease has spread from a less civilized to a more civilized community or the reverse. Syphilis started its European career as a fulminating infection and then settled down to the more chronic type which we know today. Judging by contemporary accounts, measles seems to have carried a much higher mortality in the sixteenth century than in the eighteenth or nineteenth. Yet in the nineteenth century, syphilis, probably, and measles, certainly, regained their ancient virulence when introduced into hitherto uninfected peoples. Thus the causative organism of the disease had probably not become weakened or attenuated by its long association with a particular group of individuals, for it showed all its former power when implanted into an isolated community. It is more likely that the community itself developed a partial and inherited resistance to the onslaught of the organism; although the individual had not developed full resistance and so was liable to acquire the disease, he had been endowed by his mother with a partial resistance which enabled him to struggle more successfully against the organism and so cause his illness to be less severe. This maternal resistance may be sufficient to afford absolute protection during the first months of life. This is not the whole truth, for there is evidence that strains of bacteria can and do change their character, but generally a disease, when introduced into a community which has never met it before, will prove more severe than in a community which is accustomed to it. Thus 'the state of civilization' is of only minor importance; a new infection will be more lethal to an unprotected community whether introduced from a higher or a lower level of civilized life.

Much of this chapter will be devoted to the group of diseases known as acute infections, which have sometimes been called 'zymotic' diseases. They are diseases of the crowd and cannot have flourished in the primitive races of small, scattered settlements; their origins lie in the earliest large concentrations of the human species, in such places as the Nile Valley, Mesopotamia, India and China. The reason is that the organisms of an acute infection can only transfer from one person to another when the disease is active; they can only be transmitted by the actively sick human. This is in contradistinction to such an illness as typhoid fever which can be

114

disseminated by an infected but not actively sick carrier, and to diseases which can be spread by third parties such as the typhus-bearing louse or a flea from the plague-stricken rat.

An attack of one of these acute infections will confer immunity from second attacks upon the sufferer, generally, though not always, for life. A person who is immune not only cannot acquire the disease, but also cannot transmit it, because the disease can only be transmitted when active. The disease is never entirely absent from the community; there will always be sporadic cases and minor outbreaks with a large scale epidemic every few years. For the continuance of these acute infections requires a reservoir of people who have never suffered from the disease; the number of susceptible children will be at a minimum after a severe, widespread epidemic and, equally, the chances of transmission from one individual to another will be at their lowest. As more children are born, the number of those who are susceptible will obviously rise and so will the chances of large-scale transmission from sporadic cases; thus the conditions for an epidemic will in time be present.

Historically, large epidemics of childhood diseases have been of great economic importance in European development. When the disease has been a lethal one, as in the case of smallpox, recurrent epidemics attended by a high mortality have prevented a rapid increase in population. A poverty-stricken people, breeding unchecked, will produce families of a size which the wage-earning parents cannot support; if the process is uncontrolled, then the non-productive element of the population will reach such a proportion that it cannot be fed by the productive. This state would have been reached in the past had it not been for the natural check imposed by a high disease mortality in infancy and early childhood.

Such is the pattern of acute infection when it is endemic in a community, but the picture becomes entirely different when the infection is suddenly introduced into a community which has not previously experienced it. Since no one has suffered the disease, no one has developed an immunity. Thus the acute infection will not be primarily a disease of childhood; all ages will be at equal risk. Further, since a partial resistance usually exists among even those who are still susceptible to an endemic disease but cannot exist among the individuals of a disease-free community, the acute infection may and probably will be more vicious in its effect.

This group of childish infections, sometimes known as the acute exanthemata, consists of smallpox, chicken pox, measles, german measles and scarlet fever. All are characterized by a rash, and our forefathers had great difficulty in distinguishing one from another; it is not always easy to decide which ailment they were attempting to describe. We shall not attempt to unravel the tangled history of chicken pox, german measles, and scarlet fever; we will concentrate instead on the equally intricate story of smallpox and measles.

The earlier of these two diseases to be described is undoubtedly smallpox, but its antiquity is a matter for argument. Many of the older school of medical historians held that smallpox was known in Greece and Rome, some being of the opinion that the plague of Athens (430 B.C.) and the plague of Galen (A.D. 164-180) were smallpox. But this view is not generally accepted. In 1901 Paul Kübler made the pertinent observation that there is no known classical statue or caricature which portrays a pock-marked face and no mention of any such disfigurement by medical or lay authors. The typical pock mark could hardly have escaped notice.

Another theory holds that smallpox originated among the Huns and was introduced into China in A.D. 49. Certainly the first recognizable description of the disease was written by Ko Hung, a Chinese who lived A.D. 265-313. But probably the most likely focus of infection is to be found in India, where the protection of the goddess Shitala has been invoked against smallpox from very early times. In Europe, Gregory of Tours described what was undoubtedly a smallpox epidemic in A.D. 581. Four hundred years later, in about A.D. 980, we have the first record of special isolation hospitals for smallpox cases; this was in Japan and there is also mention of a very interesting form of treatment: hangings of red cloth were used in the Japanese hospitals, and in 1314 were also recommended by the Englishman John of Gaddesden, whose manuscript was printed at Pavia in 1492. This 'red treatment' persisted as a folk remedy for many centuries and was given a semi-scientific status by the Danish pioneer of light therapy, Niels Ryberg Finsen, in 1893. Finsen used red light by means of a screen which excluded the ultra-violet rays, but the treatment was of little value.

The most authoritative early account of smallpox is by the Persian physician Abu Bakr Muhammad ibn Zakariyya, commonly known as Rhazes, in the tenth century A.D. Rhazes was the first to distinguish between measles and smallpox, but he believed them to be differing manifestations of the same disease. Belief that there was an affinity between the two persisted until 1784.

Smallpox certainly existed in Europe, Asia and Africa from the tenth century onwards, but the nature and history of the disease during the earlier part of this period is obscure. It does not seem to have been so widely prevalent and was certainly not so lethal as in the eighteenth and early nineteenth centuries. Many contemporary writers regarded measles as a more dangerous sickness, and a quite common diagnosis was a combination of both 'small poxe and mesles'. As we have already pointed out, 'great pox' referred to a major skin eruption, such as occurred in the early days of syphilis; the term 'small pox' may have been applied to a collection of ailments characterized by a skin rash and might have included the lesser cutaneous eruption of syphilis as well as chicken pox and german measles. The same muddled terminology appears in France and Germany: in France *'la grosse vérole'* meant syphilis, while smallpox was *'la petite vérole'*; in Germany the word *'Blattern'* was applied to syphilis during the sixteenth and seventeenth centuries, but by the eighteenth century had come to mean smallpox.

There is another complication. 'Smallpox' exists in three forms: *Variola major* or true virulent smallpox; *Variola minor* or alastrim, a comparatively mild form; *Variola vaccinae*, the disease primarily of cattle known as cowpox. An attack of any one of these forms will protect, at least temporarily, against the other two; this is the basis of vaccination.

The question arises of whether the disease of the fifteenth and sixteenth centuries was the mild alastrim rather than the virulent smallpox. Ralph Major implies that such was the case in India; he holds that, although a mild form of smallpox existed in India at least as early as the fifth century A.D., the first Indian description of virulent smallpox is not found until the sixteenth century. The fate of the Aztec civilization during the thirty years 1518-48 not only illustrates what happens when a new disease is introduced to an unprotected community, but also suggests that the European population was already protected from virulent smallpox by attacks of the minor form.

Spain established colonies in the West Indies during the early years of the sixteenth century. On 18 November 1518, Hernando Cortez sailed from Cuba with a force of 800 mixed Spaniards and Indians. He landed on the coast of Yucatan, made his way inland, and received friendly messages and presents from the Emperor Montezuma of Mexico. Continuing his voyage down the coast, he founded the city of Vera Cruz, assured the continued loyalty of his doubtful troops by burning the ships so that they had no means of return, and marched inland to Tlascala. Here he concluded an alliance with the natives after some hard fighting. Cortez then set out for Mexico City with his small force and 1,000 or so of his new Tlascalan allies, brilliantly avoiding a trap set for him by Montezuma at Cholula.

Cortez reached the capital on 8 November 1519. The city of some 300,000 people stood in the middle of a great lake and was approached by three causeways of solid stone, one of them six miles long. For a time he maintained good relations with Montezuma and treated him as a ruler. After learning of an attack upon Vera Cruz, apparently instigated by Montezuma, Cortez imprisoned him, forced him to acknowledge the overlordship of Spain, and fined him a considerable quantity of gold. Six months later Cortez learned that a rival Spanish expedition, under Panfilo de Narvaez, was striking inland from the coast with the apparent intention of restoring Mon-

tezuma to power. Cortez left one of his officers, Pedro de Alvarado, in command of the capital and hastened with a mere
handful of men to intercept Narvaez, defeating him in a night
attack at Cholula. Fourteen days later there came news that
Alvarado was fighting off a rising in Mexico City. Cortez
hastened back; on his arrival in the capital on 24 June 1520,
he found himself faced with a general revolt of the Aztec
nation under the leadership of Montezuma's brother. Montezuma himself tried to pacify his people, but was killed either
by a shower of stones hurled by his subjects or by the Spaniards. The small Spanish force was unable to hold the city,
and Cortez fought his way out with the greatest difficulty,
losing half of his small army in the retreat. After a heroic
struggle the remnant succeeded in reaching Tlascala.

By the end of 1520 Cortez had received some Spanish reinforcements, recruited an army of 10,000 Tlascalans, and built
a number of small ships. Having made alliances with the
intervening tribes, he dug a canal from Tlascala to the lake
of Mexico City, to bring up his boats, and began a siege of the
city in April 1521. Cortez himself commanded the boats with
a task force of 300 men; after defeating a large fleet of canoes
he made landings on the causeways and attacked the city. An
attempted general advance of his army was repulsed with
many casualties. The city finally fell, after a stubborn
defence, on 13 August 1521. The victorious Spaniards found
the houses filled with dead. Cortez had enlisted an ally more
potent than his small Spanish army or his Tlascalan friends.

When, in May 1520, Panfilo de Narvaez left Cuba on
his voyage to Mexico, he took with him a number of Negro
slaves; it will be remembered that African Negroes had been
sent from Spain to the West Indies in the early years of the
sixteenth century. Some of these Negroes fell ill on the voyage
to Mexico and at least one of them was landed while still sick.
In the language of the Indian population of Mexico, the disease from which he was suffering became known as 'the great
leprosy'. But it certainly cannot have been true leprosy and is
extremely unlikely to have been yaws or syphilis, for the rate

of spread was much too quick for anything except an acute infection. There is little doubt that it was smallpox.

But it was more lethal than the smallpox known in six-teenth-century Europe. Within a space of less than six months hardly one village remained uninfected in the known regions of New Spain. The mortality was appalling. The infection must have been carried by the Tlascalans to Mexico City and introduced at the time of the abortive general advance. For, when Cortez entered the city, he found that nearly half of the inhabitants had succumbed to the infection. The same rate of mortality was general throughout New Spain; it has been estimated that nearly half of the native population died in this first epidemic.

Eleven years later, in 1531, a second epidemic devastated Mexico and this, too, is known to have been introduced from Spanish ships. The native Mexicans called this second epidemic 'the small leprosy'; possibly the adjective 'small' refers to the extent of the mortality rather than to the nature of the disease. In 1545 there came a third outbreak, also introduced by ship; 150,000 are said to have died in Tlascala and 100,000 in Cholula. There were further visitations in 1564 and 1576; by 1595 smallpox, mumps and measles were causing much sickness among the native population. In all, some $18\frac{1}{2}$ million of the total population of 25 million were destroyed.

There is no evidence at all that any of these diseases had existed in New Spain before the coming of the Conquista-dores. The initial epidemic may have been caused by a chance case of virulent smallpox introduced by a Negro or it may be that the milder form of smallpox, alastrim, underwent a change to the virulent type when implanted into the un-protected community. In either case the Spaniards, who were obviously relatively immune to the disease, would have been at least partially protected by previous exposure to the milder alastrim, the European type of smallpox in the sixteenth century. Whatever the explanation, there is no doubt that im-ported disease played as great a part as the Spanish con-querors in the destruction of the Aztec race, if not a greater one. Thereafter Mexico remained one of the few reservoirs of virulent smallpox. As late as 1947 a traveller from Mexico introduced a limited outbreak of the virulent type into New York.

In Europe during the whole of the sixteenth century smallpox remained a comparatively mild illness and did not attract much attention until the beginning of the seventeenth century. In 1629 the first Bills of Mortality for London listed smallpox under a separate heading; the number of deaths averaged about 1,000 a year until 1680, the total population of the city being between 300,000 and 400,000. Queen Mary died during an epidemic in 1694. By the end of the seventeenth century smallpox had become the most common disease of childhood, but infants and young children often developed the mild form; mortality was much higher among older children and adults. This was well-recognized; in 1685 Samuel Pepys and John Evelyn visited a friend at Bagshot in Surrey and were much interested to see her young children running in and out of their brother's room so that they might 'take' a mild attack.

But, at the end of the century, smallpox started to change its nature. From being a comparatively mild though common disease of childhood, it became the most lethal illness of the very young. Throughout the eighteenth century smallpox destroyed more young children than any other disease, with the possible exception of infantile diarrhoea. In one English provincial town, 589 children died of smallpox between 1769 and 1774; of these, 466 were under three years old and only one over ten. During much the same period in Berlin, 98 per cent of all deaths from smallpox were of patients below the age of twelve. In London about 80 per cent of deaths were of children under five. The contemporary physician Rosen von Rosenstein stated that smallpox every year killed one-tenth of all Swedish children in their first twelve months of life.

By now the virulent type of disease had become endemic in Europe, causing a number of deaths every year and flaring into great epidemics at all too frequent intervals. Although primarily a disease of childhood in Europe, it could still affect all ages when introduced into a susceptible community. In

1789 an extensive and fatal epidemic occurred among the aboriginal natives of New South Wales, Victoria and South Australia. This visitation resulted from a chance introduction by a stricken British ship and only the Aborigines were attacked. The long sea voyage militated against infection by means of a single case, and it was not until 1829-30 that a second severe epidemic occurred; in this case white settlers were affected as well as Aborigines. Presumably no long series of cases occurred in a visiting ship between 1789 and 1829; during this half-century some of the white settlers had produced a second generation who had no resistance.

The nineteenth century saw another and an ultimately far more important change. Deaths seem to have decreased slightly from about 1796. In 1837-40 the last of the really great epidemics visited England; thereafter, a fair amount of smallpox occurred, both sporadically and in epidemics, but it tended to be localized, a disease of cities and particularly of the London slums. The age distribution also changed. Out of the total smallpox deaths in London the percentage occurring in the first five years of life fell from 80 per cent to 62 per cent in 1851-60, 54 per cent in 1861-70, and 30 per cent in 1871-80. Charles Creighton, one of the leading historians of English epidemic disease, wrote in 1894:

> It first left the richer classes, then it left the villages, then it left the provincial towns, to centre itself in the capital; at the same time it was leaving the age of infancy and childhood.

He added that smallpox, although it might have surprises in store, was a dying disease at the end of the nineteenth century.

Creighton did not believe that this decrease of virulence owed anything to compulsory vaccination. Yet vaccination is one of the greatest of medico-social advances, for it was the first attempt to defeat a disease upon the national scale. Further, it was the first attempt to protect the community as opposed to the individual. It is the first and outstanding example of

Man's endeavour to wage massive battle against his age-old enemy, pestilence.

Even the most ignorant of witch-doctors must have observed that some diseases are by nature chronic and others acute, that a patient may fall victim to the same disease quite frequently and that other diseases will only attack the patient once in his lifetime. Thus the phenomenon of acquired immunity, though not expressed in that term, has been common knowledge for centuries. Reason would suggest that, if a dangerous disease does not strike the same individual more than once, a mild attack of that disease is wholly desirable. Since it was known that disease passed from one person to another, it would also be reasonable to suppose that to protect an individual he should be placed in contact with the mildest type of case available. This idea was quite common in folk medicine. The crude method of purposeful contact suggested a refinement, the transplantation of some tissue or secretion from a mildly infected patient into an individual who has not developed the disease.

This is 'inoculation' or, in the case of smallpox 'variolation', and has been used for over 1,000 years. It is known to have been practised by Chinese physicians at the beginning of the eleventh century, and is believed to have been introduced into China from India. The Chinese inoculators removed scales from the drying pustules of a person suffering from mild smallpox, ground the scales to a fine powder, and blew a few grains of this into the nostrils of the person to be protected. Inoculation was not used in Europe until smallpox began to be a very serious problem in the eighteenth century, when a Greek physician, Giacomo Pylarini of Smyrna, removed some of the thick liquid from a pustule and rubbed it into a small scratch made with a needle.

In 1713 another Greek physician, Emanuel Timoni of Constantinople, wrote an account of Pylarini's method to Dr John Woodward of London, who had it printed in the *Philosophical Transactions* of the Royal Society in 1714. This paper aroused some interest in Britain and America, but it was not until 1721 that inoculation became at all popular. In

March 1717 Lady Mary Wortley Montagu, wife of the British ambassador at Constantinople, had her infant son inoculated and described the operation in a letter home to her friend Mrs Sarah Chiswell on 1 April. In the same year she returned to England and was there in 1721 when a great smallpox epidemic caused many deaths. Lady Mary had her five-year-old daughter inoculated during this epidemic, in the presence of several leading physicians who were impressed by the mildness of the subsequent attack. The British royal family now became interested, but George I decided to take precautions before submitting his own grandchildren to the ordeal. Six prisoners under sentence of death at Newgate volunteered to be guinea-pigs on promise of reprieve; trial was next made on eleven charity school children of varying ages. So successful were the results that two royal grandchildren received treatment.

With this example, inoculation became fashionable and was fervently supported by many leading physicians in Europe. But there was a good deal of opposition, which increased when it became clear that success did not always follow. The ensuing and protecting attack of smallpox was by no means always a mild one; it has been reckoned that two or three persons died out of every hundred inoculated. Further, many people rightly suspected that inoculation, even though it might protect the individual by a mild attack, spread the disease more widely by multiplying the foci of infection. For these reasons inoculation fell into general disrepute in Europe after 1728.

But the story had taken a different turn in the American colonies, which were first infected with smallpox during the latter part of the seventeenth century by British settlers in Maryland. From there the disease spread to Virginia, Carolina and New England. Because of the lesser density of population, it never became so prevalent as in eighteenth-century Europe, but it was one of the greatest killers and aroused equal fear. In April 1721 ships from the West Indies brought smallpox to the port of Boston, Massachusetts. The famous minister, Cotton Mather, a Fellow of the Royal Society, had read of Timoni's experiments with inoculation in the *Philosophical Transactions* and suggested to the Boston physicians that trial should be made of the method during this quite severe epidemic. Only one, a doctor named Zabdiel Boylston, showed interest. Boylston first inoculated his six-year-old son and two Negro slaves; by September he had inoculated thirty-five people with satisfactory results and with no deaths. He was accused of spreading smallpox and on one occasion had a narrow escape from lynching, but lived to see general acceptance of inoculation in America before he died in 1766. For, in 1738, a very severe epidemic of smallpox ravaged the town of Charleston in South Carolina and Dr James Kilpatrick claimed that the high mortality had ceased after mass inoculation. It was about this time, or a few years before, that Benjamin Franklin lost his only son from smallpox and became a fervent advocate of inoculation. Another supporter was George Washington. During the War of Independence Washington urged inoculation of his troops and special hospitals were set up for the purpose.

In 1743 James Kilpatrick came to London from Charleston, wrote an account of the 1738 epidemic and emphasized that inoculation had been outstandingly successful; he also described an improved method. Through his enthusiasm and because of the greatly increased prevalence of smallpox in the latter half of the eighteenth century, inoculation came back into favour throughout Europe. During this period the most successful and sought-after inoculators were Robert Sutton, his son Daniel and Thomas Dimsdale. In France, Voltaire became an ardent protagonist; it was he who aroused the interest of Catherine the Great of Russia. In 1768 Catherine invited Dimsdale to visit Russia, where, after successful experiments on the lower orders of society, he inoculated the Empress, her sons and many members of the imperial court. Dimsdale received a truly regal fee for his services: £10,000, with an additional £2,000 for expenses, an annuity of £500, diamond-studded miniatures of Catherine and her sons, and the rank of baron.

There is no doubt that in Europe, and especially in Britain, inoculation could be an actual danger to the community because smallpox was more common in cities, where the density of population made isolation of inoculated cases difficult. For this reason, inoculation was almost entirely confined to the wealthier classes who could be isolated in the home or in a special hospital. The problem was not so great in America, because a lower density of population made precautions against spread of the inoculated disease more feasible. Washington's provision of inoculation hospitals for his troops was reported in England. Right at the end of the eighteenth century English physicians, such as John Coakley Lettsom, strongly urged the foundation of similar institutions for inoculation of the poor. In 1798 the introduction of a new and safer method of immunization made the provision of such hospitals unnecessary.

The method of variolation or inoculation necessitates implanting smallpox into the subject. The resultant illness is smallpox, even though it may be only a mild attack, and it can be transmitted from one person to another. Vaccination, however, necessitates only that a smallpox-like disease of animals, cowpox, be implanted into the human. Cowpox is caused by a virus very similar to that of smallpox; it will protect the individual against smallpox proper for a time, but, because the person protected is suffering from cowpox and not smallpox, he cannot transmit smallpox to a second subject. This is why inoculation or variolation is dangerous to the community, whereas vaccination is safe.

The fact that cowpox protects against smallpox has probably been part of folk-knowledge for centuries, but the first known deliberate use of cowpox as a means of protection is in 1774. In that year a severe epidemic of smallpox attacked the small village of Yetminster in Dorset, and a number of the inhabitants were inoculated. Benjamin Jesty, a farmer and cattle-breeder, was aware of the popular belief that cowpox would protect against smallpox, for two of his servants had suffered from cowpox and nursed several smallpox patients without catching the disease. Jesty took some of the matter or lymph from the pustules of an infected cow and rubbed it into scratches made with a darning needle on his wife and two sons. None of them developed smallpox but Jesty met with a great deal of criticism for making inhuman experiments upon his family. Fifteen years later, in 1789, a doctor named Trowbridge, who practised in the Dorsetshire village of Cerne, inoculated both of Jesty's sons with matter from a smallpox pustule; in both cases nothing happened. Another instance of deliberate cowpox vaccination is known from Holstein: in 1791 Peter Plett, tutor in a landowner's family, vaccinated his employer's children. Three years later an epidemic struck the village of Schonwaide, where this family lived, and the subjects of Plett's experiment are said to have been the only children in the village to escape infection.

These isolated experiments did not influence the course of medicine. The experiments of Edward Jenner are in a different category. Jenner was a doctor in practice at Berkeley in the dairy-farming county of Gloucestershire. In 1796 a dairymaid named Sarah Nelmes attended his surgery because she had developed the pustules of cowpox upon her hand. Jenner knew of the widely-held belief that cowpox protected against smallpox. He took some of the lymph from one of the pustules and scratched it into the skin of a boy, James Phipps. Several weeks later he inoculated young Phipps with matter from a smallpox pustule and found that he failed to develop the disease in any form. For two years Jenner continued with his vaccination experiments. He gave cowpox the name of *Variola vaccinae*, and showed that it was unnecessary to use lymph from infected cattle. 'Humanized cowpox vaccine', that is, lymph from cowpox pustules on human skin, is equally effective. Thus Jenner was able to counter the widespread objection to inoculation with an animal disease. In 1798 Jenner published his historic (and now very valuable) pamphlet *An Inquiry into the Causes and Effects of the Variola Vaccinae, a disease discovered in some of the Western Counties of England, particularly Gloucestershire, and known by the name of Cowpox.*

Jenner's work excited considerable interest. Confirmation of his findings came from Henry Cline, a well-known surgeon of Guy's Hospital, and from George Pearson, a physician of St Thomas', who later opened the first public vaccination centre. In 1799 M. Woodville of the Smallpox Inoculation Hospital in London made a fairly extensive trial of vaccination with satisfactory results. It is reckoned that 100,000 people had been vaccinated in England alone before 1801. In 1807 the Royal College of Physicians of London was ordered by government to examine and report upon the method. The College concluded that vaccination produced an illness milder and less dangerous than inoculation, that vaccinated persons who contracted smallpox were seldom seriously ill, and that vaccinated persons did not spread infection. For these reasons the College strongly recommended the practice, while admitting that in some instances it failed to protect against smallpox.

In 1840 inoculation of smallpox was made illegal in Britain; the same Act provided for free vaccination at will. Vaccination of infants became compulsory in England and Wales by an Act of 1835; ten years later compulsion was extended to Scotland and Ireland. In Germany compulsory vaccination was introduced in 1874 and the law contained the wise provision (never enforced in Britain) that re-vaccination must be performed at the age of twelve. Holland required compulsory vaccination only when the child started school. In the United States of America, the first man to practise vaccination (1799) was Professor Benjamin Waterhouse of the Harvard Medical School. Waterhouse is said to have secured his supply of cowpox lymph from England, but how a living and active virus survived the Atlantic crossing in 1799 is rather mysterious. He first vaccinated seven persons, among them his own children, and then inoculated all seven with smallpox; in every case smallpox failed to develop. Waterhouse became an enthusiast and found an active supporter in President Thomas Jefferson, who had eighteen members of his own household vaccinated. The first American establishment for free vaccination was founded in New York by Valentine Seaman in 1802.

Vaccination is a controversial topic. But something virtually put an end to European and North American smallpox by the time of the First World War, and it is difficult to escape the conclusion that that 'something' was vaccination.

But there are two mysterious points. First, although only seven cases of smallpox were notified in 1917, no less than 14,767 were notified in 1927. What had happened during this decade? In 1919 a quite large local epidemic of smallpox occurred in Norfolk and Suffolk, but the illness was very mild and rarely fatal. In 1920 an outbreak in Lancashire caused eighty-three known cases but not a single death. Thereafter this very mild form of smallpox, or alastrim, rapidly increased until the peak of 1927 and then as rapidly decreased until only one case of smallpox was notified in 1935. This form seems to have been a recrudescence of the smallpox that existed before the seventeenth century; it became widely disseminated throughout the world and is now the prevalent type except in India, China and parts of South America.

The second point may explain the first. Is vaccination inoculation with true cowpox or are we using a very attenuated strain of the smallpox virus? Jenner was the first man to employ arm-to-arm vaccination, that is, the humanized cowpox vaccine. That early advocate of vaccination, Dr Woodville of the Smallpox Inoculation Hospital, obtained his original supply of lymph from a cow belonging to a dairy in Gray's Inn Lane, London. With this lymph he vaccinated seven persons. He then inoculated all seven with matter from a smallpox pustule, three of them *after an interval of only five days*, when they cannot possibly have developed an immunity to smallpox. He then vaccinated a first series of 200 people and a second series of 300. But he did not use lymph from a cow. All of the first 200 were vaccinated with lymph from the original seven cases, and most of these were later inoculated with smallpox. The second 300 were all vaccinated with lymph from the first 200, and many of these were also inoculated.

Describing his experiments, Woodville acknowledged that 'in several instances, the cowpox has proved a very severe disease. In three or four cases out of 500, the patient has been

129

in considerable danger, and one child actually died.' It therefore looks as though some of Woodville's patients suffered a quite severe attack of smallpox. Arm-to-arm vaccination, rather than cow-to-human vaccination, became the method of choice and was almost exclusively practised until the 1860s. The particular virus strain used by Woodville very probably persisted, certainly in London, probably in the rest of Britain (since he possessed more vaccinated patients than anyone else) and possibly in America (since Waterhouse is said to have received his first vaccine from England in 1799). The late Dr A. H. Gale believed that 'the bringing together of cowpox and smallpox virus did in some way produce a modified smallpox virus which ... gradually became safer and safer.' He added that the modern virus of *vaccinia* resembles that of smallpox rather than that of cowpox.

If Gale is correct, Woodville's original attenuated strain must also have passed to animals. One very commonly held objection to arm-to-arm vaccination is that other diseases, such as tuberculosis and syphilis, may be accidentally implanted. Acting on this belief, Negri of Naples in 1845 artificially propagated the virus in cows, initially using a humanized lymph, and thereafter employed bovine lymph for vaccination. The practise spread to France in 1866 and thereafter to most of Europe. Calf lymph began to be used in the United States in 1870; the original lymph was obtained from France and inoculated into a herd of cows on a farm near Boston, Massachusetts. This gives a basis of reason for Gale's contention.

Vaccination has done its work by changing smallpox from an endemic into an exotic disease. But vaccination often confers immunity for as little as five years; complete protection against smallpox can only be obtained by re-vaccination at stated intervals. It is intelligent for the individual to have himself vaccinated before visiting a country in which smallpox is known to occur; it is intelligent for the community to insist upon previous vaccination of an individual who comes from an infected to a non-infected country. It is essential that every person who has been in contact with a sporadic case of smallpox should be vaccinated or re-vaccinated. This requires a certain amount of detective work on the part of health officials and calls for ceaseless vigilance. Provided that vigilant watch is maintained, there is no reason why smallpox should ever again become a major problem.

The early histories of measles or morbilli and smallpox are similar; while it is unlikely that measles did not exist in the ancient world, there is no unquestionably recognizable description of the disease until that of Rhazes in the early tenth century A.D. Confused terminology bedevils the story: morbilli is derived from the Italian *morbillo*, the little disease, in contradistinction to the plague, *il morbo*; 'mesel' is used by Chaucer and Langland to denote leprosy; 'small poxe and mesels' is a common sixteenth-century term for what appears to have been a single disease. The muddle persisted as late as the eighteenth century, and the confusion seems to have been more in terminology than in diagnosis; thus 'measles' or 'morbilli' was quite frequently applied to 'scarlatina' or scarlet fever, while 'scarlet fever' was sometimes the name given to diphtheria.

Measles probably first appeared during the Middle Ages in France; it was certainly well established as a fairly severe infection in Europe during the sixteenth century. In this connection, and when studying the history of all diseases, we must remember that the invention of printing by movable type about the year 1455 not only added greatly to ease of communication but also made it far more probable that the record would persist until the present day. The very large sixteenth-century literature on syphilis has suggested to some historians that syphilis must have been a new disease in Europe. As we have already seen, the disease in this case probably was a new one, but the existence of this literature cannot be adduced as proof; all that happened was that many authors 'rushed into print' and their books have been preserved. John of Gaddesden described smallpox and also measles; he wrote his manuscript in the early fourteenth century, but we should probably know nothing of it had it not been printed at Pavia in 1492. Thus we must not fall into the error of thinking that the sixteenth century saw the introduction of many new diseases into Europe. Many were clearly described and, because they were printed, the descriptions are known to us today, but the diseases antedate the descriptions.

By the seventeenth century physicians were beginning to distinguish measles from smallpox, and the 1629 Bills of Mortality for London contain measles under a separate heading. Not many deaths are recorded, but two epidemics occurred in 1664 and 1670, causing 311 and 295 deaths respectively. In 1674 came a more serious outbreak with 795 deaths; after this measles declined until the epidemic of 1705, which caused 800 deaths. From the beginning of the eighteenth century, epidemics became more frequent and, towards the end of the period, occurred once in about every three years. There were unusually bad epidemics, with a high mortality in 1718 and 1733. These coincided with a time of excessive gin-drinking, which has sometimes been held to blame. In so far as the parents would have been in no condition to nurse their children efficiently, gin may have indirectly affected the mortality; good nursing can greatly decrease the mortality of measles, for death does not occur from measles itself but from its complications, chiefly pulmonary or of the ear.

So far as can be judged, the type of measles encountered in the eighteenth century was generally mild. In 1785 William Heberden of London stated that it was rarely necessary to call in a doctor. In 1762 the French physician Tissot pointed out that measles rarely killed; when death occurred, it was due to some complication. Towards the end of the century the European picture changed: the disease became far more common, more dangerous and more widespread. This was the beginning of the great epoch of measles, when hardly a child in Europe escaped infection, when major epidemics occurred in every second year, when measles was one of the more common causes of death in childhood. In the twentieth century, measles apparently became less virulent but it is a better standard of living, more educated child care and smaller families, rather than medical advances in treatment, which have lessened mortality.

From the sixteenth until the beginning of the twentieth century the European has carried measles with him on all his explorations, often with devastating results. New Spain was infected quite early in the sixteenth century; some historians believe that 'the small leprosy' which ravaged Mexico in 1531 was measles rather than smallpox. In North America, wide spaces and a scattered population, with frequent immigration from Europe, produced a rather different pattern of infection. Epidemics tended to be less frequent, more severe when they occurred, and attacking people of all ages rather than young children. The first known epidemics were in Canada in 1635 and 1687. Boston was attacked in 1657 and again in 1687, the latter possibly being an import from Canada. Further epidemics occurred in 1713, 1729, 1739 and much more severely in 1740. South Carolina, Pennsylvania, New York, Connecticut and the remainder of Massachusetts were attacked in 1747 and then there was no major outbreak until 1759. This was followed by an epidemic in 1772, which was particularly severe in Boston and surrounding districts: 800 children are said to have died in Charlestown, Massachusetts. Six years later, in 1788, New York and Philadelphia were ravaged by measles. The disease followed the covered wagon, appearing first in the Mississippi valley and then in Kentucky and Ohio.

The course taken by measles in America was dictated not by the nature of the disease but by the growth and cohesion of population. Scattered communities were separately infected and a considerable time might elapse before such a community was again attacked. If the lapse of time was twenty years, then all age groups up to twenty years were at risk and the age incidence might be widened by the immigration of adults from uninfected areas. As the distance between centres decreased and communication became easier, so the chance of infection increased. Thus epidemics became more frequent until the nineteenth century, when rapid travel and greater density of population changed the pattern into one similar to that obtaining in Europe. Measles, in fact, became an endemic disease of America, never entirely absent, and reaching epidemic proportions at intervals.

But nineteenth-century speed of communication was not confined to Europe and America. Slow travel by sailing ship over long sea routes gave place to the faster steamer. Rapid contact could be made with communities which had hitherto been entirely cut off, or visited at rare intervals after months of voyage without touching land. Thus certain island communities received the full weight of an infection which they had never before experienced. Since they had never been infected, the individuals possessed no immunity, either maternal or acquired. In circumstances such as these, the disease would spread with frightful rapidity, all ages would be at risk, and mortality would be unusually high.

The most important of these island epidemics from a medical point of view is that which struck the Faroes in 1846. The Faroe islanders had already experienced measles, but no case occurred between 1781 and 1846; that is to say, no one under the age of sixty-five could have been immune. On 20 March 1846, a workman left Copenhagen, landed in the Faroes on 28 March, and developed symptoms of measles on 1 April. The population of the Faroes numbered 7,864; 6,100 fell sick of measles between the end of April and October, the number of deaths being 102. The mortality, expressed as 1.6 per cent of infected cases, is certainly not very high for those times.

The medical interest of this outbreak lies in the fact that the Danish government sent a twenty-six-year-old doctor, P. L. Panum, to deal with the situation. Panum took the opportunity of making a close study of the epidemic and much of the knowledge of measles derives from his work. He found that there is an incubation period of 13-14 days during which the patient can transmit the disease, a very actively infectious period while the typical measles rash is present, and then a non-infectious stage of desquamation or 'peeling'. Panum concluded that measles can only be carried by direct contact between individual and individual and that isolation of all known contacts is the best method of controlling an epidemic.

He also suggested that one attack of measles conferred life-long immunity, for he found that not one of the ninety-eight inhabitants who had suffered from measles in 1781 developed the disease in 1846. Panum's theory was proved when measles again struck the Faroes in 1875, for only persons under thirty years of age were attacked.

In the same year of the Faroe Island epidemic, 1846, an entirely different type of outbreak occurred among the native Indian population of the Hudson Bay Territory in North Canada. In this small epidemic, lasting for just six weeks, 145 people of all ages fell sick and no less than forty died, a mortality which can be expressed as well over 25 per cent. More recently an example occurred of what will happen when a community, previously isolated, is brought into sudden contact with a centre of endemic infection. At the beginning of the First World War, a Highland Division from the sparsely populated north of Scotland was encamped at Bedford in the south-east of England. From October 1914 until March 1915, they experienced 529 cases of measles with sixty-five deaths, a mortality of 12.3 per cent. The disease was commonest and most lethal among those men who had come from the remoter parts of the Highlands.

We cannot claim that any of the outbreaks so far described exerted a major effect upon the course of history. But the story is rather different when we consider the population tragedy which measles brought to the islands of the South Pacific in 1875. In 1872 epidemic measles developed in South Africa, spreading to Mauritius in 1873-4 and to South Australia in 1874. On 10 October 1874, the British Government annexed the Fiji group. Early in 1875 a cruiser, H.M.S. *Dido*, visited the islands. A few sailors had fallen sick of measles and some, only slightly ill, were permitted to land while still in the acutely infectious stage.

Within a little over three months, at least one-fifth and probably more nearly a quarter of the native Fijian population died; the total number of deaths in the Fiji group alone was over 40,000. The panic which developed must have been something like that attending the Black Death in Europe six centuries before. A contemporary writer, William Squire, believed that many natives died from sheer terror, others from seeking relief by immersing their fever-stricken bodies for long periods in the sea. Squire added that 'the epidemic only ceased when every person had been attacked'. From the Fiji group measles passed to all of the South Pacific island communities, with equally devastating results. It was not the only gift which civilization brought: tuberculosis and syphilis caused many deaths and helped to ruin the physique of the magnificent island races. No one knows how many died; it is widely believed that disease has reduced the South Pacific native population to about one-tenth of the number who lived in the islands a century ago.

6
Disease and the Exploration of Africa

Men have encountered and overcome terrible dangers as they have forced their way into every corner of the earth. A long sea voyage in tiny ships led the Spanish Conquistadores to a hostile terrain in South America. The vast, featureless plains and high mountain ranges of North America, inhabited by fierce Indian tribes, did not deter the pioneers in their covered wagons as they journeyed from the Atlantic to the Pacific. Geographical barriers can be overcome; fierce wild beasts are powerless before even a flintlock musket.

But it was not the larger animals that were the most dangerous; until almost the end of the nineteenth century minute creatures were the unbeatable enemy: the mosquitoes breeding in steamy swamps, the tsetse flies of the African savannahs and forests. Not dangerous in themselves, their bites injected even smaller organisms, the minute parasites which cause malaria, the virus of yellow fever, the trypanosomes which produce sleeping sickness. Tropical heat, damp and dirt provide ideal conditions for bacteria. Without strict sanitary control the water-borne diseases such as typhoid fever and dysentery sapped the energy and caused thousands of deaths among white settlers. It is the prevalence of these diseases which accounts for the fact that Africa, although colonized along its northern shore by Greek and Roman, remained almost unknown territory until the end of the nineteenth century.

The fly- and water-borne diseases so weakened expeditions that penetration of the interior became impossible; the white man's health could be maintained only when he understood the cause of his sickness and how it could be controlled. Even on the coast he lived in peril. So demonstrably unhealthy was the West Coast of Africa that many physicians, of whom James Lind is a notable example, believed that the upland interior must provide better living conditions for the white man. The practical difficulties of exploration were unsuspected. The hot river deltas, through which boats must make their way from the coast into the interior, teemed with mosquitoes and so with yellow fever and malaria. Dysentery and the enteric fevers waited all along the route. Wounds caused by thorns or other means festered and refused to heal, causing debility and often death. Trypanosomiasis affected not only men in the form of sleeping sickness, but also cattle in the disease known as nagana. Perhaps this last was the most decisive: David Livingstone wrote that the tsetse fly was 'fatal to horses and cattle and a barrier to progress'; because of nagana, the horse could not be used for transport in Equatorial Africa; all cross-country journeys had to be made on foot, goods being carried on the heads of natives.

There were many attempts to penetrate the secrets of the interior. The Portuguese, who first founded stations on the African coastal plain, explored part of the lower and middle

Zambezi River in the sixteenth and seventeenth centuries. In 1569 a party on horseback tried to strike inland in search of gold. Word was later brought back that all the horses died, while the men succumbed to disease and attack by hostile tribes. In 1788 the African Association for the exploration of the interior was founded in London. A Scottish surgeon, Mungo Park, offered his services and set out to discover the source of the Niger River. He failed, returned to Scotland, and then tried again. Park left the Gambia on 28 April 1805, having with him, 'besides Mr Anderson, Mr Scott and Lieutenant Martin, 34 soldiers, 4 carpenters, and 2 seamen, in all 44 Europeans. He did not reach the Niger at Bambakoo until 19 August, far into the rainy season, having had to traverse 500 miles of a country fertile of disease and beset with danger. Dysentery and fever had by this time made sad havoc amongst his people, for there remained alive only 11 of the whole, and on 11 October all, except 4, were dead. Whether any white man, save Lieutenant Martin, survived to perish with him at Borissa sometime in November, has not been ascertained.' Mungo Park himself had severe dysentery. He was drowned with the remnant of his party in the rapids. Their fate remained unknown for five years.

In 1816 Captain James Tuckey, R.N., tried to explore the River Congo. He took his ship as far as the rapids, where he landed a shore party which included several scientists. They found the climate 'pleasant, the thermometer seldom exceeding 76°F or being lower than 60°F, with scarcely any rain and the atmosphere dry'. Despite the favourable conditions the expedition was attacked by 'an intense remittent fever with black vomit in some cases'. Fourteen men died on land and 4 more after returning to the ship, all within three months. The dead included Captain Tuckey and the scientists. The total European mortality of this expedition can be expressed as 37 per cent.

In 1832 Major A. M'Gregor Laird penetrated the Niger delta with two ships, *Quorra* and *Albrukah*. They entered the Benue tributary on 18 October 1832. By 12 November nearly all the men were down with fever; on the 14th only one European was fit for duty. The *Quorra* reached the sea in August 1833, only 5 of her 29 Europeans having survived. *Albrukah* returned to the Niger delta in November, having lost 15 out of 19 Europeans.

Equally disastrous was the large expedition led by Captain H. D. Trotter in 1841. In all, 145 white Europeans, 25 coloureds recruited in Britain, and 133 Africans recruited in Sierra Leone, took part. They travelled in three iron-built steamboats, *Albert, Wilberforce,* and *London,* which reached a point on the Niger about 100 miles from the sea on 26 August. Fever broke out at the beginning of September 'and ceased not until it had paralysed the whole expedition'. They pushed on, but sickness became so prevalent that *Wilberforce* and *London* were sent back to the coast on 19 September, laden with their own sick and those from *Albert. Albert* steamed further up the river but was forced to return on 4 October, reaching the coast ten days later, having been on the river for nine weeks. Of the 145 Europeans, 130 fell sick of fever and 50 died. Eleven of the twenty-five British coloureds were attacked by fever, but all of these recovered. None of the 133 Africans recruited in Sierra Leone fell sick.

The fate of these expeditions—and there were many more, equally disastrous—clearly shows why the interior of Africa remained unknown territory for so long a time. The comparative sickness rate of Europeans and Africans puzzled medical men. Many theories were put forward to account for the immunity of the natives. Perhaps God had purposely arranged matters so that the African might live in peace. Or perhaps Negroes avoided fever because they were ignorant of European luxurious living. Or perhaps they had a greater capacity for perspiration and were better able to throw off the 'foul and nasty vapours' which poisoned the European body. But most medical authorities held that Africans were differently constituted. They gave a scientific, or at least a medical, basis for racism. Medical opinion held that the white man could not perform manual labour in the African climate without falling sick. Thus the white man's function was to direct and to govern; only the Negro could carry out heavy work. These vacillating and erroneous medical ideas resulted in many deaths and the abandonment of hopeful policies.

Malaria was perhaps the most generalized and dangerous of the African diseases. It is caused by a minute protozoon, a plasmodium, of which there are several strains. *Plasmodium malariae* or *P.vivax* is more common in Europe and America; *P.falciparum* is the prevalent African parasite. A European who had developed a resistance to the type of malaria caused by *P.vivax* would still be susceptible to the type caused by *P.falciparum*. The parasites have a complicated life history, multiplying asexually in the human bloodstream and completing their sexual life-cycle in the body of the mosquito. Very briefly, the parasites are injected into the human by the bite of a female *Anopheles* mosquito, go through various phases, take up their lodging in the red blood cells, feed on the haemoglobin and burst the envelope of the cell. In so doing, they release toxic products formed by the digestion of haemoglobin. These toxins cause the typical malarial attack, a cold stage, hot stage, and stage of sweating. Signs of malaria appear about a fortnight after being bitten, the onset varying slightly according to the number of parasites injected. This incubation period is the time taken for the rapidly dividing parasites to form a sufficient number—several hundreds in every cubic millimetre of blood—to affect health. It takes seventy-two hours for the parasite to invade a red blood cell, grow to fill it, divide into six to twelve new individuals and burst the cell wall, thus releasing toxins into the bloodstream. As all the parasites injected by one mosquito bite are in the same stage of development and as they adhere fairly rigidly to their developmental timetable, attacks of malaria occur at regular intervals. Thus we have the old term 'tertian ague', an attack occurring every seventy-two hours; that is, every third day. 'Quartan ague' is caused by another plasmodium which has a longer developmental cycle. The predominant African type, caused by *P.falciparum,* is known as malignant or sub-tertian malaria; it is a far more dangerous disease in which death may occur quickly. If death does not occur during the first attack, and the patient is regularly reinfected, his subsequent attacks may be little more than chills and a slight fever. Untreated quartan or tertian malaria rarely kills by its own direct action; it is a chronic infection that causes increasing ill-health and renders the sufferer more liable to attack by other diseases and less able to resist them. The chief reason for this ill-health is the chronic anaemia resulting from the parasite's destruction of the haemoglobin contained in the red blood cells, the iron-containing pigment essential for carrying oxygen to all parts of the body. If malaria attacks a community on a large scale, it will cause a mass decline in vigour.

We can trace this mass effect from very early times. Malaria seems to have been common in the neighbourhood of Athens during the fifth century B.C. In Rome, where there was a steady decline over a period of four centuries, there were recurring plagues of malaria. It is likely that malaria produced an anaemic community suffering from nation-wide ill-health, with a predisposition to attack by other illnesses, a falling birth rate, physical and mental lassitude, and a consequent lowering of morale. The malarial parasite continued to infest Greece on a large scale until comparatively recently, producing a 100 per cent infection of the population in some districts. The same is true of Italy, where the district of the Pontine Marshes was particularly notorious. Nineteenth-century travellers to these regions remarked on the feebleness of the population, their squalid life, and their miserable agriculture.

Malaria seems to have attained its widest distribution in Europe during the seventeenth century, when very few countries, if any at all, escaped infection. Oliver Cromwell, born in the English Fenland, suffered from malaria all his life and died on 3 September 1658 of 'a tertian ague'. At postmortem, his spleen was found to be 'a mass of disease and filled with matter like the lees of oil'. This is a fairly common termination of malaria: the spleen is enlarged and may either be ruptured by a quite minor accident or suffer a spontaneous haemorrhage into its substance. In the first case, the patient will bleed to death unless operation is performed;

in the second, the blood clot may become infected and form an abscess which will cause death from toxaemia. The disease was relatively common in England until 1840 and then rapidly declined until, by 1860, it had become a rarity except in the Isle of Sheppey off the Kentish coast. The present writer, while going through the old case-notes of his hospital, has found details of a patient who had never travelled abroad, yet acquired malaria in 1874; he lived in the Plumstead Marshes, a waterlogged area bordering the River Thames, only ten miles south-east of the City of London. This should remind us that the *Anopheles* mosquito is still found in England, as in many other malaria-free countries. It is the malarial parasite and not the mosquito, still capable of carrying the parasite, which has disappeared.

Until the seventeenth century malaria was treated in the same manner as other fevers; indeed many physicians only recognized two types of fever: 'intermittent' and 'continuous', a classification which led to disaster when applied to the prevalent fevers of Africa. Purging, starvation and bleeding were the accepted remedies and must have hastened the end of many unfortunates who suffered from the anaemia of malaria. Early in the century, the bark of a tree was shipped to Spain from Peru and was found to be effective in the treatment of malaria. For many years it was thought that the bark, cinchona, took its name from the Countess of Chinchon, wife of the Governor of Peru, who had been cured of an obstinate fever by taking this native remedy, and who as a thank-offering had distributed large quantities freely to the citizens of Lima and taken a supply back to Spain. The true story is much less romantic. The Peruvian Indians applied the name *quina-quina* (bark of bark) to a tree—myroxlyon—which yielded Peruvian balsam. Balsam of Peru became so popular a remedy in Europe that supplies ran short and adulteration with similar barks was common. A bark from the cinchona tree was frequently used. The two barks were thus prescribed indiscriminately for many years until it was at last found that cinchona, and not the much vaunted myroxlyon, gave good results in the treatment of malaria. In 1820 two French chemists, Pierre Pelletier and Joseph Caventou, extracted the active alkaloid, quinine, from cinchona bark. Quinine is lethal to the malarial parasite, can be used in the cure of malaria, and is also fairly effective in preventing the disease if taken regularly so as to maintain the necessary level in the blood.

Quinine is one of the classical examples of empirical treatment; no one knew the cause of the disease or why the drug worked, but it did work. Unfortunately it had very unpleasant side-effects when taken in sufficiently large doses: vomiting, headache, rashes, disturbances of vision and hearing. The latter was the most noticeable; quinine-takers often suffered from such severe tinnitus or 'singing in the ears' that they were quite deaf. A better and more modern drug is a derivative of quinine, chloroquinine. Just before the Second World War an entirely new drug, mepacrine hydrochloride or atebrin, was introduced. This could be used as a prophylactic to prevent malaria and as a suppressant, to suppress the effects of developed malaria. During the campaigns in Burma and New Guinea, mepacrine proved most successful and practically stamped out the lethal form called blackwater fever. But this drug, too, had unpleasant side-effects. Not only did it stain the whole skin yellow, but it caused vomiting and, sometimes, cerebral excitement. More recently U.S. servicemen in Vietnam have been treated with single doses of pyrimethamine and sulphormetoxine, and this has proved very effective. Recent outbreaks of malaria in the U.S. have been traced to soldiers who have neglected prophylactic treatment while in Vietnam, and a number of single cases have occurred in Britain, among other countries, because travellers to malarial areas have thought it unnecessary to take precautions for a few days' stay. The *Anopheles* mosquito persists and can still become infected with the parasite.

For many years malaria, particularly the virulent African type, was confused with yellow fever, often known as Yellow Jack because it was a common cause for quarantining ships and a ship in quarantine flies a yellow flag. Yellow fever is caused by a virus, injected through the bite of another type of mosquito, *Stegomyia* or *Aëdes*. It is a far more acute disease than malaria, some of the distressing and dangerous symptoms being high fever, jaundice, vomiting, intractable diarrhoea, suppression of urine, and profound exhaustion. One attack protects the patient for life. Thus, in areas where the disease is endemic, a considerable mass immunity develops and, as in the case of measles, some maternal immunity is conferred upon children. Yellow fever therefore tends to be a less severe illness among native populations than when introduced to communities which have never experienced it. This is why Yellow Jack became so feared by seamen who plied between Africa and America in the eighteenth and nineteenth centuries; one case occurring on board ship might easily wipe out the whole crew.

The original habitat of yellow fever is not certain. It was probably taken from Africa by ship to America and the West Indies early in the sixteenth century. Some epidemiologists believe the reverse, that the disease originated in Central America and was introduced to Africa. They base their theory on the fact that the first well-documented outbreak occurred in Barbados, St Christopher, Guadeloupe, Havana and Yucatan in 1647-8. For a long time it was thought that the first African epidemic was that described by John Peter Schotte at St Louis de Senegal in 1778. More recently it has been found that John Williams, a surgeon of Kingston, Jamaica, having described a West Indian outbreak, went on to write:

I do not apprehend this fever is what we call a local disorder; for I have seen it on the coast of Africa and am well informed that in the River Benin they have a bilious or yellow fever acuter than what it is here, at the time of the expedition to Carthagena; the person seized with this fever dying there in less than twenty-four hours.

John Williams had been a surgeon on a Guineaman, that is, a slaving ship plying between Guinea and the West Indies.

The date of his own African experience is not clear but the Carthagena expedition took place in 1740-1.

The most interesting point in Williams's account is that he tried to differentiate between yellow fever (*Synochus atrobiliosa*) and malaria (bilious remittent fever). Williams may have been the first practitioner to understand the difference, and the reason for his understanding was his experience in both Africa and the West Indies. The very prevalent and severe type of malaria found in West Africa, often associated with the lethal blackwater fever (characterized by the passing of dark urine, due to the massive breakdown of haemoglobin by malarial parasites), probably obscured the presence of true yellow fever on the African coast. Williams's views aroused great hostility in Jamaica (which seems to have been proud of its reputation for yellow fever) and resulted in a duel with his chief antagonist, Dr Parker Bennet, in which both men were killed.

Whether yellow fever originated in Africa or America, it became a common disease in many parts of the world during the seventeenth, eighteenth and nineteenth centuries. Particularly severe epidemics occurred on the eastern seaboard of America, extending as far north as Halifax, Nova Scotia, which experienced a bad outbreak in 1861. New York suffered in the 1690s, while a hundred years later, in 1793, Philadelphia was ravaged by an epidemic which must have equalled in its horrors a visitation of bubonic plague. At least one tenth of the population died between April and September. Morale fell to a very low level; Howard W. Haggard in *Devils, Drugs and Doctors* quotes:

> While affairs were in this deplorable stage and the people at the lowest ebb of despair, we cannot be astonished at the frightful scenes that were enacted, which seemed to indicate a total dissolution of the bonds of society in the nearest and dearest connections. Who, without horror, can reflect on a husband deserting his wife, united to him perhaps for twenty years, in the last agony; a wife unfeelingly abandoning her husband

146

on his deathbed; parents forsaking their only child without remorse; children ungratefully flying from their parents and resigning them to chance, without an enquiry after their health or safety?

A shining light in this dark tale is provided by the behaviour of Philip Syng Physick, sometimes called the Father of American Surgery. Physick left America for London to study under the great John Hunter; Hunter pressed him to remain as his assistant but he preferred to return. Only twenty-five years old, he had just settled in practice in Philadelphia when the epidemic started. Physick tended his patients devotedly until he himself was attacked. He recovered but never regained his previous strength. Later he was appointed surgeon to the Pennsylvania Hospital and professor to the University.

The conquest of malaria and yellow fever is of great importance. The two may be considered together as knowledge of both diseases clearly depends upon appreciation of their insect spread. In 1877 (Sir) Patrick Manson, then of Hong Kong, demonstrated that embryos of minute worms, called *Filaria*, which are one of the causes of elephantiasis, were ingested at night from human blood by the *Culex* mosquito, developed in the insect's body, and were transmitted when the mosquito again bit a human. Manson's theory was not believed but, in 1881, Carlos Finlay of Cuba made the similar suggestion that yellow fever was spread by mosquito bites, although he could produce no definite evidence. Meanwhile in 1800 a French army surgeon stationed in Algeria, Alphonse Laveran, had discovered malarial parasites in the red blood corpuscles of infected patients by microscopical examination. They were also observed by an Italian, Camillo Golgi, who noted a difference between the parasites of tertian and quartan malaria.

In 1894 Manson, now working in London, met Ronald Ross, a young surgeon on leave from the Indian army, and showed him Laveran's malarial parasites in a blood film. Manson told Ross that he believed the parasites developed in 'some suctorial insect', just as the ova of *Filaria* worms were incubated in the body of the *Culex* mosquito. Ross made a long investigation, and eventually, on 20 August 1897, discovered malarial parasites in the stomach of the *Anopheles* or Spotted-Winged Mosquito. His findings were confirmed in the following year by Giovanni Grassi of Rome, who also showed that the female *Anopheles* is the only kind of mosquito capable of transmitting malaria. The life-cycle of the parasite was gradually worked out. In 1900 infected mosquitoes, sent from Italy to London, were allowed to bite Ross's son, who developed malaria. A control experiment was equally successful: three of Ross's assistants went to live for some months in specially mosquito-proofed huts in the Roman Campagna and failed to develop malaria.

These findings renewed interest in Carlos Finlay's theory of yellow fever. Walter Reed was an army surgeon who had studied under the great bacteriologist, William Welch of Baltimore. In 1900 Reed joined Carlos Finlay in Havana with two assistants from Baltimore, James Carroll and Jesse Lazear, to form a Yellow Fever Commission. Lazear and Carroll allowed themselves to be bitten by the *Stegomyia* or Tiger Mosquito. Both developed yellow fever; Carroll recovered but Lazear died within a few days. Walter Reed carried on the work and, having proved the association between mosquitoes and yellow fever, was able to suggest methods of control which virtually freed Havana from yellow fever within a year. Reed died in 1902 and was succeeded at Havana by William Crawford Gorgas, who had himself fallen ill of yellow fever early in his career while an army surgeon in Texas. It was Colonel Gorgas who was in command of the dramatic campaign against malaria and yellow fever during the building of the Panama Canal.

The long voyage from the Atlantic to the Pacific could only be reached by the notoriously dangerous passage round Cape Horn at the extreme tip of South America. In 1879 Ferdinand de Lesseps started to investigate the possibility of digging a canal across the narrow Isthmus of Panama, following the line of a railway which had already been constructed.

De Lesseps estimated that the work could be completed in about eight years but he encountered immense difficulties and his project ended in May 1889. For a time the Panama route was entirely abandoned and a longer canal through Nicaragua proposed. In 1904 the United States became actively interested in the Panama route and recommenced digging in 1907. Seven years later the Americans completed their fifty-mile long canal (deep Atlantic water to deep Pacific) and the first ship, the U.S. War Department vessel *Ancon*, passed through on 15 August 1914.

The three-year period 1904-7 is the critical time in the history of the Panama Canal. Some of de Lesseps's difficulties had been financial, but the terrible sickness rate and mortality among his workmen proved the most serious problem. Mosquitoes abounded in the lakes and undrained swamps through which the canal must pass. Malaria and yellow fever caused havoc. It is said that a labourer died for every sleeper laid on the Panama railway; the death rate among workers on de Lesseps's abortive canal amounted to 176 per 1,000. In 1904, when the Americans decided to start work again, William Gorgas was put in charge of the health arrangements. One preventive measure advocated by Walter Reed in Havana had been isolation of all yellow fever patients in mosquito-proofed rooms; this, with a campaign against the *Stegomyia* mosquito, had been the reason for success. Gorgas proposed a similar programme, but he found it difficult to convince the authorities that mosquitoes, and not dirt, were the cause of malaria and yellow fever.

After a hard battle, he at last persuaded the government-run Canal Commission to take action on the Havana lines. Sanitary brigades were organized on a large scale and for two years conducted an intensive campaign against the mosquito. Special buildings were prepared for workers and officials, all of them protected by fine copper-gauze netting. Stagnant water was drained off and pools filled in wherever possible. Very good results followed spraying of choked drainage channels with weed-killer; this not only allowed a freer flow of water but destroyed the resting places of adult mosquitoes.

When drainage proved impossible, pools were regularly sprayed with kerosene to kill mosquito larvae. By 1907, when intensive work on the canal started, yellow fever had already been beaten and the incidence of malaria had fallen very considerably. The last fatal case of yellow fever occurred in 1906; by 1914, when the canal was completed, mortality from all causes in the Panama Canal Zone had fallen from 176 per 1,000 in the 1880s to only 6 per 1,000. This compared with an over-all death rate of 14 per 1,000 throughout the United States and 15 per 1,000 in London. Colonel Gorgas, through whose efforts this magnificent triumph was achieved, organized the medical services of the United States Army in the First World War.

The terrible African trypanosomiasis or sleeping sickness is caused by a minute parasite, known as a flagellate, belonging to the genus *Trypanosoma*. It is carried by the tsetse fly, a member of the species *Glossinia*, of which there are many varieties infesting different parts of Africa. There are two distinct forms of trypanosomiasis, the African and the South American. The latter, sometimes called Chagas's Disease after Carlos J. R. Chagas who first described it, is caused by *T.cruzi*, carried by a species of louse, and is only found in Brazil and Venezuela.

African trypanosomiasis occurs widely between latitudes 12°N and 25°S; that is, in the area lying roughly between the Gambia River on the north-west coast and the Limpopo River on the south-east. Thus the area embraces the whole of the Great Central Plateau and all Equatorial Africa. Two types affect man: the *gambiense* type, which is widely distributed in west and central Africa, and *rhodesiense*, which occurs in eastern and central districts. The two types are carried by different varieties of tsetse fly, which differ in their habits. Those which carry the *gambiense* type thrive in shade and high humidity, so are only found in hot, damp river bottoms with abundant vegetation. The carriers of *rhodesiense* live in open, scrub-covered country. This differing habitat implies that few parts of central Africa are free from trypanosomiasis.

Gambiense is a disease of the humid forest regions, *rhodesi-ense* of the dry savannahs.

The bite of a tsetse fly is very painful. The spot bitten swells up and then subsides, much like the bite of an ordinary horse-fly. If the tsetse is infected, the bitten place will again become painful and swollen about ten days later. This swelling is sometimes called the trypanosomal chancre on the analogy of the chancre produced by syphilis. The trypanosomes invade the patient's bloodstream within two or three weeks, when the generalized disease process begins. The clinical picture varies with the type.

Gambiense is the more chronic. There are irregular bouts of mild fever and the glands, particularly at the back of the neck, become enlarged with a distinctive rubbery feeling. The bouts of fever become longer, sometimes lasting for as much as a week. The liver and spleen enlarge. After some months, the central nervous system is affected. The patient complains of severe headache and his behaviour changes: lethargy often alternates with outbursts of senseless anger, sometimes accompanied by physical violence. There is reversal of the normal sleep rhythm: the patient suffers from insomnia at night but is somnolent by day. He develops tremors and paralyses of the limbs, loses his appetite, and starts to waste away until reduced to little more than a skin-covered skeleton. Gradually he sinks into a coma, which deepens until he dies.

Rhodesiense is generally a more acute illness. The fever is much higher and more constant; the patient is seriously ill within only a few weeks of being infected and death often occurs quickly from a direct effect upon the heart. If progress of the illness is less acute, the final stages will be much like those of *gambiense*: tremors of the limbs, increasing drowsiness and coma.

Sleeping sickness is undoubtedly a disease of African origin, but the first accurate account in 1803 was by an English doctor, Thomas Masterman Winterbottom of Cuba, who observed it in slaves imported from Africa. Winterbottom later worked in Sierra Leone. David Livingstone, the great missionary-explorer, described the tsetse fly in 1857 and stated that horses and cattle died from its bite. The disease of horses was known as nagana or stallion sickness. Livingstone treated infected animals with arsenic; his treatment must have been empirical for the cause was then unknown, but arsenical preparations were the first hopeful medicines to be used in human sleeping sickness.

The incidence of sleeping sickness rose considerably and epidemics became more frequent in the last years of the nineteenth century, because new trade routes were opened and there was increased movement in the hitherto almost static equatorial belt. Nagana became more common at the same time. In 1894 (Sir) David Bruce, an army medical officer, arrived in Natal to investigate the problem of nagana. He was accompanied by his wife, who actively assisted him in his work. They examined the blood of all infected horses and cattle brought to them and discovered a parasite which became known as *Trypanosoma brucei*. Bruce showed that the parasite was conveyed to animals by the bite of tsetse flies, thus confirming and expanding Livingstone's observation of 1857.

In 1901 John Everitt Dutton, a doctor working in Gambia, found a trypanosome in the blood of human patients suffering from sleeping sickness; hence the name *T.gambiense*. Dutton's work was ended prematurely in the following year when he died while investigating another insect-borne disease, relapsing fever, on the Congo River. In 1903 a large outbreak of human sleeping sickness occurred in Uganda; David Bruce went to investigate with his wife and a team which included the famous Italian expert on tropical diseases, Aldo Castellani. Castellani was particularly interested in the nervous symptoms shown by the patients, the tremors and paralyses, the alternating violence and drowsiness. He examined the cerebro-spinal fluid, contained between the two membranes which enclose the brain and spinal cord, and he there found a minute parasite. Bruce, informed of this, turned his attention to the blood of sleeping sickness patients and discovered similar parasites. These were identical with the trypanosomes which he had discovered in the blood of cattle suffering from nagana. All the bits of the puzzle fell into place. Bruce showed beyond question that both nagana of animals and sleeping sickness of humans are due to a trypanosome and that the trypanosome is carried by tsetse flies. Spread could be controlled by restricting the movement of infected people and cattle, and by destruction of the flies.

Unfortunately it was not quite so easy as that. Control of the *gambiense* type is comparatively simple, for the vector fly will only thrive in humid shade. Stripping the hot, damp river banks of their vegetation destroyed the breeding grounds and caused the fly to disappear. But *rhodesiense* is carried by the fly of the arid, scrub-covered savannahs. It infests domestic cattle and, incidentally, causes a serious problem by limiting production of meat and milk, so helping to cause the terrible fatal disease that affects fast-growing children, known by the Ghanaian name of Kwashiorkor, which is due to a deficiency of high-grade protein foodstuffs and is still a problem in undernourished countries. Some control can be obtained by limiting the movement of cattle and by clearing wide areas of scrub. This method derives in part from the folk-knowledge of African herdsmen: the fly is only active by day and the herdsmen found that they could safely drive cattle from one grazing ground across scrub country (the 'fly belt') to another ground at night. Another source of infection is wild game and the movements of these animals cannot be entirely controlled. Although wild animals act as a reservoir and spread the disease, they are not themselves affected. It has been suggested that encouragement of game in large reserves might provide a more ample supply of protein foods than domesticated cattle.

Until the early 1920s treatment of the disease, whether *gambiense* or *rhodesiense*, was practically useless. A drug, atoxyl, and very large doses of tartar emetic, given intravenously, were often prescribed. European travellers to fly-infested districts were advised to wear gauze veils over the face and neck, gloves, and long trousers tucked into boots—an uncomfortable kind of attire in a hot and sticky climate. About 1922 the German firm of Bayer introduced a useful drug, the arsenical compound tryparsamide. Much more recently a complex organic urea compound, suramin, and the arsenical preparations melarsopropol and trimelarsen, have proved effective. Another drug, pentamidine, is used prophylactically; one injection will protect against the *gambiense* type for six months. These measures, combined with intensive warfare against tsetse flies, have brought human sleeping sickness under control.

We turn from the diseases that are carried by insects to three of those that are carried by water: typhoid fever, dysentery and cholera, which although not an African disease is relevant to our story. The enteric group—typhoid, paratyphoid and food-poisoning—are caused by bacilli; dysentery is caused either by a bacillus or by an amoeba, a primitive unicellular organism. The enteric fevers and the dysenteries, although they produce different patterns of disease, can be considered together, for their chief interest lies in the fact that they are primarily caused by a contaminated water supply. Epidemics have been traced to other sources—infected milk, butter and ice-cream are examples—but, until very recently, water has been most frequently to blame.

Since contaminated water is the cause, the diseases must be of great antiquity; the first epidemic must have occurred when the first infected man defaecated and washed himself at a point up-river from the place where his community drew its drinking supply. Until the late nineteenth century, it was impossible to distinguish typhoid and paratyphoid from the more lethal typhus fever, because both were called 'continuing fevers'. The dysenteries, characterized by painful diarrhoea and passing of blood, were more easily diagnosed. Good accounts of the symptoms are given in the Ebers Papyrus and in the works of Hippocrates; we have already indicated that the sickness which smote the Philistines, described in Samuel I, may have been dysentery rather than the more usually accepted bubonic plague. Water-borne diseases, now commonest in tropical countries, were found in the past, and by no means the remote past, wherever men shared a common water supply without sanitary precautions. In such circumstances, risk was greater in high densities of population; hence the terrible epidemics of typhoid fever in early nineteenth-century industrial towns; hence, probably, the 'summer diarrhoea' which was one of the chief causes of infant mortality until sixty years ago.

Typhoid and dysentery were so common among troops upon active service that they have been called campaign diseases. Until very recently, armies were so prone to infection by drinking contaminated water that sickness invariably produced a greater death roll than did wounds. Disease is no respecter of persons; we can gain an idea of the prevalence of water-borne disease by considering the fate of some of the English monarchs who led their armies in person. William the Conqueror died from a ruptured ulcer in the large bowel, a late result of typhoid fever; King John probably died from the same cause although his end is romantically attributed to 'a surfeit of peaches and new cider'. 'Peaches and cider' could hardly cause death by themselves but might easily precipitate a diarrhoea violent enough to rupture a weakened bowel wall. Edward I died of dysentery and so did the hero of Agincourt, Henry V. Edward the Black Prince, son of Edward III, also succumbed to an enteric disease, probably dysentery, and his early death may have affected the course of history, for his weak young son, Richard II, came to the throne during the land and labour crisis following the Black Death, one of the more difficult periods in the development of English society. Coming to more recent times, Albert the Prince Consort, husband of Queen Victoria, died of typhoid fever in 1861; his son, the future Edward VII, nearly lost his life from the same disease ten years later.

The English soldiers at the battle of Crécy in 1346 were so riddled with dysentery that the French called them the breechless or bare-bottomed army. Reliable statistics give a grim picture of disease in nineteenth-century warfare. About 1 million men were engaged in the American Civil War of

1861-5. In the Northern Armies 93,443 men were killed on the battlefield or died of wounds; almost exactly double that number, 186,216, died of disease. This figure does not include 24,184 who perished from unknown causes. Of the total who died from disease, 81,360 deaths were due to typhoid fever and dysentery. Accurate figures are not available for the Southern or Confederate Armies, but it appears certain that typhoid caused more deaths than in the Northern.

The Boer War of 1899-1901 is of considerable interest because the organisms of typhoid fever and dysentery had been discovered and measures for prevention, including anti-typhoid inoculation, were available. By then typhoid was recognized as a water-borne disease; it was known that filtering or boiling water would render it safe. But the British soldier did not take kindly to water and sanitary discipline. The Berkefelde and Pasteur filters soon became clogged and did not yield water freely; in the hot climate of South Africa boiled water was slow to cool. Typhoid developed in the army early in the war, during the hurried march to Bloemfontein along the Modder River. The soldiers could not be prevented from drinking water straight from the river although it was known that typhoid was prevalent in villages upstream. About 400,000 troops in all were sent to South Africa, the field army numbering 200,000 at any one time. From February 1900 until the end of 1901, 6,425 died in battle or from wounds, while 11,327 died of disease. The total of typhoid patients in the army amounted to 42,741.

The Russo-Japanese War of 1904-5 was the first war in which wounds took a greater toll than sickness; the Russians claimed that only 7,960 soldiers died of disease out of a total of 709,587 engaged. The figure is probably an underestimate, but foreign observers agreed that the standard of health in the Russian armies was excellent. The Russians did not release the number of battle casualties, which are thought to have been considerably less than the Japanese, who lost 58,357 men by enemy action and 21,802 by disease; of the latter 5,877 succumbed to typhoid and dysentery. Typhoid fever was as prevalent in Manchuria as in South Africa. The greater success of both Russian and Japanese sanitary control depended upon strict discipline. Troops were forbidden to drink unboiled water, care was taken to provide constant supplies of hot water for making tea, and troops were, so far as possible, never billeted in villages.

From dysentery and typhoid we pass to the last, and most important, of our water-borne diseases, Asiatic cholera. Here is another mystery. Why did cholera confine itself to India for at least 2,000 years and then suddenly erupt in world-wide pandemics? No one can give the answer. There are some who hold that the story is not true, that cholera was one of many disputed diseases which have struck various countries from the earliest times; if this be so, and there is no evidence in favour, then cholera equally mysteriously disappeared from the European scene at about the time of the Renaissance and did not reappear until 1826.

The first recognizable mention of cholera occurs in the writings of Hindu physicians about 400 B.C. Almost 2,000 years later, in 1498, the expedition led by Vasco da Gama was stricken by a virulent epidemic, thought to have been cholera although there is no good evidence as to its nature. It is certain that British garrisons of the East India Company had lost thousands of men from cholera by the end of the eighteenth century, the most deadly area being the Ganges delta. The holy city of Benares, a place of pilgrimage, stands on the Ganges; it is probable that the vast concourse of pilgrims, who themselves suffered heavily, contaminated the water upstream and so infected the whole of the river complex which drains into the Bay of Bengal.

1817 is the fateful year. A ship brought the infection to Arabia, whence it spread to Persia, Turkey and Astrakhan in southern Russia. The strange point is that there was simultaneously an eastern spread to Malacca, Siam and, later, to Japan. By 1826 a great pandemic covered Arabia, Persia and the whole of European Russia. Poland, Germany, Austria and Sweden became infected before 1829. The first English cases appeared at Sunderland in October 1831, and the whole of Europe and the British Isles were invaded in 1832-3. Quebec and New York were infected in 1832 and the disease then spread slowly south to Mexico and Cuba.

This was the first of six great and two lesser pandemics which occurred between 1817 and 1902. We know why the pandemics died out but why did they never occur before 1817? There was a considerable traffic between Europe and the Portuguese, French and British trading posts in India from the sixteenth century onwards. The British had a station at Calcutta from 1653 and were firmly established in Bengal after Clive's victory at Plassey in 1757. Bengal was a centre of cholera; merchant ships of the East India Company plied regularly between India and London; London was just as insanitary in the eighteenth century as in the early years of the nineteenth. Yet no case of cholera is known to have occurred in England until 1831. It has been argued that the Napoleonic wars gave an immense impetus to ship-building, that fast sailing boats so shortened the time of travel that an epidemic aboard ship could no longer burn itself out during the voyage. But infection does not seem to have been by ship. Initially cholera may have reached foreign ports adjacent to India by this means, but thereafter there was a slow relentless spread across land masses rather than by sea. It is probable that there was a change in the behaviour of the causative organism.

In England, by January 1832 cholera was rife in the Tyneside but did not appear elsewhere until April. John Snow, a medical apprentice of Newcastle-on-Tyne, was sent by his master to help in an outbreak at the nearby Killingworth colliery. Here Snow made a number of observations which were to form the basis of his great work when England was again attacked by cholera seventeen years later.

In 1840 another outbreak started in Malacca and spread slowly, inexorably round the world, reaching Europe, North Africa and North America in 1848-9. This was the most serious of all the pandemics and did not cease until 1856-8. It was particularly severe in France, where over 140,000 people died. In Britain the death roll was 52,000; Italy lost about 24,000. The pandemic coincided with the Crimean

War of 1854-6 (although some epidemiologists hold that this was a separate outbreak) and all the armies suffered severely. The French, British and Piedmontese lost about 18,000 from cholera alone out of a total of just over a quarter of a million men engaged.

Cholera reached London in December 1848 but did not become general until June 1849. John Snow, now medically qualified, had moved to the capital, where he became the first specialist anaesthetist in the world but retained his early interest in epidemiology. One of the worst affected districts was an area around Golden Square, quite close to where he lived. He resumed the study of the disease which he had begun in 1832. While investigating the outbreak at Killingworth colliery, Snow had come to the conclusion that cholera was not carried by bad air nor necessarily by direct contact. He formed the opinion that the intractable diarrhoea, unwashed hands and shared food played a large part in spreading the disease. He inquired into the habits of miners and received one illuminating reply:

The average time spent in the pit is eight to nine hours. The pitmen all take down with them a supply of food, which consists of cake, with the addition, in some cases, of meat; and all have a bottle, containing about a quart of 'drink'. I fear that our colliers are no better than others as regards cleanliness. The pit is one huge privy, and of course the men always take their victuals with unwashed hands.

Snow followed up this idea in the cholera-ridden slums of London and, incidentally, threw a light on the terrible conditions which added so much to the prevalence of disease. Two of his examples will suffice:

The bed linen nearly always becomes wetted by the cholera evacuations and the hands of persons waiting on the patient become soiled without them knowing it; they must accidentally swallow some of the excretion, and leave some on the food they handle or prepare, which has to be eaten by the rest of the family, who, amongst the working classes, often have to take their meals in the sickroom; hence the thousands of instances in which, amongst this class of the population, a case of cholera in one member of the family is followed by other cases; while medical men and others, who merely view the patients, generally escape.

In the asylum for pauper children at Tooting, one hundred and forty deaths from cholera occurred amongst a thousand inmates. The children were placed two or three in a bed, and vomited over each other when they had cholera. Under these circumstances, and when it is remembered that children get their hands into every-thing, and are constantly putting their fingers in their mouths, it is not surprising that the malady spread in this manner.

Here was the answer to the spread of cholera among the poor, but how did it reach the houses of the rich? Snow took his reasoning a stage further:

There is often a way open for it to extend itself more widely, and to reach the well-to-do classes of the com-munity; I allude to the mixture of cholera evacuations with the water used for drinking and culinary purposes, either by permeating the ground and getting into wells, or by running along channels and sewers into the rivers from which entire towns are sometimes supplied with water.

In 1849 the houses around Golden Square were not supplied by pipes. The residents drew their water from sur-face wells by means of hand-operated pumps. A severe out-break of cholera occurred at the end of August in a limited area centred on Golden Square, about 500 deaths occurring in ten days. In Broad Street, a road close by, the epidemic took an explosive form, breaking out suddenly on the night of 31 August-1 September and dying down after 3 September. A few cases had occurred before this date and a few occurred afterwards.

John Snow obtained permission to examine the registers. He found that 89 deaths had been registered in Broad Street during the week 27 August-2 September. There were 6 in the first four days, 4 on Thursday 31 August, 79 on 1 and 2 September. He investigated 83 deaths which had occurred in the last three days, and found that all except 10 of the dead people had lived close to a pump in Broad Street. Five of the 10 would have been expected to draw their water from a nearer pump, but preferred the Broad Street supply. Three more of the 10 were children who went to a school close to the pump; 2 were known to have regularly drunk water from it and the third was thought to have done so. The remaining 2 of the 10, wrote Snow, 'represent only the amount of mortality from cholera that was occurring before the irruption took place'. He investigated the water-drinking habits of the 69 people who had lived close to the pump and found that 61 had drawn their supplies from the pump while 6 had not. He concluded that, bearing in mind the large epidemic already raging in the district, 'there had been no particular outbreak or increase of cholera, in this part of London, except among the persons who were in the habit of drinking the water of the above-mentioned pump-well'.

The Board of Guardians of St James's parish, in which Broad Street lay, met to consider the critical situation on 7 September. John Snow attended the meeting and gave his evidence. According to the classical story, the frightened Guardians demanded of him what measures were necessary to prevent further outbreaks. Snow replied shortly: 'Take the handle off the Broad Street pump.' 'In consequence of what I said,' wrote Snow, 'the handle of the pump was removed on the following day.' No more 'irruptions' occurred in Broad Street.

Snow traced the pipe-lines of various water companies and showed that water supplied by one company was infected by cholera while that from another company serving the same district was not; he also found that certain houses served from an innocent source were infected by cess-pools overflowing into cracked earthenware water pipes, and argued that the cause of disease 'the *materies morbi*' must be capable of multiplying and so must resemble living material. Snow did not discover the true cause of cholera, the micro-organism, but he came very close to the truth. He proved beyond question that cholera is a water-borne disease and his evidence started a train of events which, in the end, controlled the great epidemics of cholera, dysentery and typhoid.

Improvement in living conditions led to a vast diminution in water-borne disease. At the end of the nineteenth century, the majority of European and North American cities were as clean as Rome had been in the first. Cholera virtually disappeared from western Europe and North America after 1874. The last great pandemic started in India in 1891 and spread to Siberia and European Russia, reaching St Petersburg in August. A coincident series of bad harvests produced terrible conditions in Russia and the disease did not die out until 1896. Hamburg was also infected by contaminated water from the Elbe, but the twin city of Altona entirely escaped because it received water from a clean source. Small ship-borne outbreaks occurred in some ports of England, France, Spain and Italy, but no serious epidemics developed. Cholera remains a problem in India, where it kills about 100,000 people a year. In 1961 a new strain of cholera organism, known as *el tor*, broke out of its home in the Celebes Islands to reach the Philippines. In 1963 *el tor* reached Korea and China. From 1964 to 1965 it spread through India, Saudi Arabia and Egypt. In 1966 it reached Iran (Persia) and in the summer of 1970 was reported on the Russian Black Sea coast, in the Caspian district and in Turkey. Antibiotic treatment has greatly reduced mortality and a new vaccine, prepared in the laboratories of the Johns Hopkins Medical School, is said to be effective for up to six months.

Typhoid fever and dysentery have also been brought under control. There are still many infected parts of the world and protective inoculation of persons visiting such localities is essential. It is probably true to say that water is bacteriologically safe in all European countries; if a visitor there spoils his holiday with a gastro-intestinal upset and that upset is due to drinking water, it is usually because the water contains minerals to which his alimentary tract is unaccustomed. Nearly all recent outbreaks of typhoid in developed countries can be traced to immigrants, refugees, or returning visitors from infected places. Typhoid poses a special problem because the organism can sometimes be carried in the bowels of a healthy person; if such a carrier is employed in the kitchens of a large institution, he or she may spread disease. Tracking down and immunization of carriers is an essential duty of public health administration.

Conquest of fly- and water-borne diseases made the colonization of Africa possible. For nearly 400 years European traders bought African slaves and shipped them first to Europe and then to the Americas. But the trader only inhabited the narrow coastal plain; he obtained his slaves from native dealers who themselves made forays into the interior. Because the European could not penetrate the interior, he exerted no direct influence upon the native inhabitants. During the early part of the nineteenth century the slave trade was brought to an end after years of propaganda and struggle. Traders still exploited the natives but no longer dealt in human lives. Missionaries and doctors, battling against immense difficulties, forced their way inland. As knowledge of the cause of disease increased and as, in particular, quinine became more readily available, they met with greater success. Most notable of these devoted men was David Livingstone who, from 1841 until his death on 1 May 1873, founded mission stations, preached to the natives and treated their diseases, and explored large areas of equatorial Africa. His exploratory work was continued by the American Henry Morland Stanley who, despatched by the *New York Herald* to search for

Livingstone after his reported death in 1869, found him alive but reduced almost to a skeleton on 28 October 1871. Disease had most certainly not yet been conquered. Both Livingstone and Stanley almost succumbed to attacks of malaria and dysentery on many occasions, and not one of the mission stations founded by Livingstone survived for more than a few months.

The true importance of Livingstone and Stanley in the story of Africa lies not in what they did, but in the enthusiasm which their examples inspired. They were the first in a long line of later nineteenth-century pioneers who stimulated international interest in the potential opportunities of Africa. Until 1875, in which year Stanley journeyed down the Congo River, the only European powers established in Africa were Great Britain, Portugal and France. The Portuguese claimed sovereignty over 700,000 square miles, but effectively controlled only 40,000. The French, almost confined to the northern seaboard, held 170,000 square miles and the British, largely in the south, held 250,000. The total area 'ruled' by Europeans amounted to 1,271,000 square miles, about one-tenth of the continent. Apart from the large desert area of the Sahara, roughly half of Africa—the greater part lying in the tropical zone—was entirely inhabited and ruled by native tribes.

The Franco-Prussian war of 1870-1 greatly affected the future of the continent. Victorious Germany became ambitious for overseas dominions; defeated France saw her own hope of renaissance in an enlarged colonial empire. The struggle for African colonies was precipitated by an initially generous movement on the part of Leopold II of Belgium. In September 1876 Leopold summoned representatives of all European powers to a conference in Brussels, the object for discussion being the exploration, exploitation and civilization of Central Africa. Delegates to this conference were not representative of their governments, who gave no official support. The conference decided to set up an International African Association with its headquarters in Brussels. As a result of international jealousy and lack of co-operation, the Association failed and the venture became purely Belgian. The Congo Free State came under the personal sovereignty, rapidly approaching the personal ownership, of Leopold II.

Leopold's rule very soon aroused hostility. The Congo River, which Stanley had shown to be a practicable waterway from its deep estuary on the coast for 1,000 miles into the heart of Africa, was an attractive geographical feature. Other countries were not slow to see the material advantages of opposition to Leopold's unenlightened rule. Portugal made renewed claims, traditional rather than valid. The French became suspicious of Belgian penetration. In January 1879 Stanley received an appointment as accredited agent of Leopold II in the Congo Free State; he established trading stations and entered into treaties with native chiefs along the south bank of the Congo. In 1880 Savorgan de Brazza, acting for France, made treaties and founded stations along the north bank, in an endeavour to link up with Timbuktu, the theoretical southern outpost of the French colonial empire in North Africa. In 1884 Germany announced her annexation of a long stretch of the west coast together with the hinterlands of Togo and Cameroon. The British who had lagged behind except in South Africa, now formally declared their sovereignty over the Niger delta, Lagos and Sierra Leone. The great land-grabbing operation had clearly got out of control and would inevitably lead to large-scale warfare unless some kind of international agreement could be reached. The Berlin Conference of powers, opened on 15 November 1884, decided that possession by a European country of any part of Africa must be effective to be valid and that all signatory powers must be notified of the intention to annex any part of the continent. The ominous phrase 'spheres of influence' appeared for the first time in this treaty. The major partition of Africa occupied slightly less than a quarter of a century. By 1914 nearly 11 million square miles had passed into European possession; only 613,000 remained independent.

There were only three independent states at the outbreak of the Second World War: the Union of South Africa, Egypt and the Republic of Liberia, which had originally been founded by American abolitionists as a home for freed slaves. By 1962 twenty-eight African states had become voting members of United Nations. Within the space of twenty-three years almost the whole population of Central Africa acquired the rights of self-government and self-determination. But the real change has been far more rapid; there are many Equatorial Africans who have hurtled from a Stone Age civilization into the Atomic Age within a lifetime. We can gain some idea of this headlong speed of advance by estimating the length of railroads in the Africa of 1934, at a time when rail was beginning to give way to the automobile in Britain and America. In the whole of Equatorial Africa there existed only 318 miles of track and the total mileage, including that of 'white' South Africa, was 42,750, just double that of Britain at the same date. The equivalent figure for Europe and Russia is 235,719. Africa, hardly touched by the horse or the Railway Age, passed directly from pedestrian transport to the car and aeroplane. This continent is, in fact, the seat of a vast technological and social experiment. No one can usefully prophesy what the future holds or what the outcome of the experiment will be. The difficulties are derived not least from the sheer speed of change. This is the sense in which the danger of infection which existed until the last quarter of the nineteenth century, and the rapid conquest of disease that we have seen in the past seventy years, may well have posed one of the greatest problems of the future.

7
Queen Victoria
and the Fall
of the Russian
Monarchy

Victoria, Queen of Great Britain and Empress of India, is at first sight a most unlikely candidate for the honour of bringing Lenin and his Bolshevik party to power in Russia. A monarch among monarchs, to whom alone the title of 'The Queen' was respectfully accorded by her reigning colleagues, she seems to have purposefully followed a policy of linking the thrones of Europe into one great family by marriage. Yet she unwittingly played a large part in the tragedy which destroyed the mightiest of European autocracies, the House of Romanov of Russia.

Her fateful mission in history was to transmit the hereditary or genetic disease known as haemophilia A to her numerous progeny. Haemophilia is the lack of a specific protein in the serum or liquid part of the blood; if this protein is absent, clotting will not take place. Since minor bleeding normally stops because the blood clots, a person suffering from haemophilia is in danger of bleeding to death from trivial cuts or bruises. The defect seems to have originated in Queen Victoria or her mother, for there is no record of any earlier blood abnormality in the family. One of her four sons, Prince Leopold, died as the result. Of her five daughters, three transmitted haemophilia to their children or grandchildren. The worst history is that of the youngest, who married Prince Henry of Battenberg. Two sons of this marriage died of the disease; a daughter, Ena, married King Alfonso XIII of Spain; two haemophiliac sons of this marriage died, aged twenty and thirty-one.

Victoria's third child and second daughter, Alice, was born in 1843 and married Louis IV, Grand Duke of Hesse-Darmstadt. There were two sons of the marriage, of whom one died of haemophilia at the age of three. Of the five daughters, one died of diphtheria when a child. The eldest was the maternal grandmother of the present Prince Philip, Duke of Edinburgh; the second married Grand Duke Serge of Russia; the third married Prince Henry of Prussia; and the fourth daughter, Alix, married Nicholas II, Autocrat, Tsar and Emperor of All the Russias, thus bringing Queen Victoria's haemophiliac gene into the Romanov family.

These hereditary factors or genes were first described by a Roman Catholic monk, Gregor Mendel, who experimented with the growing of various types of peas in the abbey garden of Brunn in Austria. His findings, buried in the pages of an obscure journal, attracted no attention when they were published, after ten years of experiment, in 1866. Thirty years later, three botanists in three different countries had the same idea; during their researches they found that Mendel had already done similar work and that his conclusions were correct.

Mendel had discovered that tall peas will not always produce tall offspring when sown, but short and tall varieties in a regular pattern. The reason is that when a tall breed is crossed with a short breed, the next generation will always be tall, but these 'tall peas' contain a 'short pea' element. Mendel postulated that the 'tall' and 'short' element must always be double. Thus a *true tall* strain would contain the two elements or factors for tallness, TT; while a *true short* strain would contain two factors for shortness, tt. If a true tall pea is crossed with a true short pea, the hybrid will contain one factor from each parent and so will have the constitution Tt. If two of these Tt hybrids are now crossed, the progeny may receive any possible combination of the factors Tt x Tt; if there are four offspring, the most likely pattern will be TT, Tt, tT, and tt. That is, a quarter of the progeny will be truly tall, half will inherit an equal factor of tallness and shortness, and a quarter will be truly short. Mendel's attention was really aroused because his peas did not produce the pattern which might be expected: one tall, two medium, and one short. Three of the plants were tall and only one short. Tallness is a dominant factor; the element for tallness T will always override the element for shortness t. Thus, all Tt and tT plants will be tall but, when one Tt plant is crossed with another Tt plant, a quarter of the progeny will have the constitution tt and will therefore be short. In 1905 William Bateson, working on the hybridization of sweet peas at Cambridge, gave to Mendel's hereditary factors or elements the name of 'genes'.

These genes, partly derived from the father and partly from the mother, decide the physical appearance of the child and the basic manner in which he or she will react to environment. Man is derived from a single female cell, the ovum, and a single male cell, the sperm. Both cells contain a nucleus; each nucleus contains a material, chromatin, which is visible under a microscope as fine, tangled threads. When the ovum is fertilized by the sperm, the two nuclei fuse to form a single cell. The billions of cells in an adult are all ultimately derived from this single cell. Thus the original cell will transmit equal elements of both male and female to the two cells into which it divides and this process will continue through all stages of growth. Before the fertilized cell divides, the tangled filamentous chromatin coalesces to form a number of roughly X-shaped bodies, the chromosomes. These chromosomes carry the genes of inheritance.

Microscopical studies have confirmed Mendel's postulate that the factor or element contained in the individual is always doubled (TT or Tt, for instance) and that only half of this factor is transmitted by each parent to the offspring. In man, the female egg cell and the male sperm each contain twenty-three chromosomes, and the fertilized cell therefore contains forty-six. This figure is almost but not entirely constant; for instance, the type of mental defective known as a mongol has an extra chromosome, making 47 in all. The number of chromosomes remains constant with each cell division in all members of the human race, but the size and shape of the chromosomes differ, and this difference affects the nature of inheritance. As it is the chromosomes which bear the genes, and as chromosomes bear different genes, and as only half the parental chromosomes are transmitted to the child, it is extremely unlikely that a child, deriving twenty-three gene-bearing chromosomes from one parent and twenty-three from the other, will exactly resemble either parent. It is also extremely unlikely that there will be no resemblance, but the resemblance is never exact; only in the case of identical twins, formed from the splitting of a single fertilized cell and therefore genetically identical, will there be any difficulty in telling one individual member of a family from another.

This familial resemblance can be traced back, by studying portraits, for a number of generations. Often a marked peculiarity of feature occurs in every generation over a period of centuries; like the drooping Hapsburg lip and narrow chin. But, if we could obtain a full-length photograph of the primitive Hapsburg who existed in 1,000,000 B.C., it is extremely unlikely that we should find much resemblance to the Hapsburgs of Austria who lived in the twentieth century A.D. The differences would be greater than could be explained by the constant infusion of fresh genes by marriage. Face and body would in fact bear little resemblance to *any* human of the present day.

This is because the genes themselves change or mutate, and it is this mutation of genes which has, in the course of millions of years, produced Man from his ape-like ancestor. Such changes are essential to the orderly process of evolution; they enable a creature to adapt itself to a gradually changing environment and to a more complex life. But sometimes things go wrong; the mutant gene produces an undesirable trait, which may take the form of disease. True genetic disease is not by any means common because if the disease limits the viability of the strain in which it occurs, then that strain is likely to die out completely in the course of several generations.

A few malformations and diseases are known to be caused by genes. One example is achondroplasia, failure of the cartilage to form bone at the growing ends of the long bones, which produces the type of dwarf often to be seen in circuses. Another striking one is the unpleasant disease known as Huntington's chorea, which causes progressive mental deterioration accompanied by continuous involuntary twitching movements. It was first fully described in 1872 by an American physician George Huntington, who attended several patients in Long Island. Some of these patients belonged to families treated by Huntington's father and grandfather, who had started practice in Long Island in 1797. Huntington was thus able to trace the families back; he showed that the disease—that is, the mutant gene—existed in a family of immigrants from Bures, a small village in Suffolk, who landed at Boston in 1630. The violent twitching and mental symptoms aroused suspicion and caused some of those affected to be accused in the notorious Salem witch trials of 1692. Huntington's chorea is a rare example of a genetic disease which persists because, although incurable, it most commonly appears in middle age. Thus there is time for children to be born before onset, and about half of these will be affected. In one case, the unbroken line could be traced back to an immigrant through twelve generations.

Porphyria is an interesting genetic disease and one which may have exercised some effect upon the course of history. The name 'porphyria' means 'purple urine' and refers to the most obvious sign, occasional passing of urine which turns a purplish brown colour on standing. The first appearance of the disease is usually in the second or third decade of life, and it takes the form of sudden attacks associated with abdominal pain and constipation, local nervous symptoms such as a hypersensitive skin, rheumatic pains, and mental disturbance. Through the investigations of Dr Ida Macalpine and Dr Richard Hunter, King George III of Great Britain and Hanover has become the best-known sufferer from this ailment. Long thought to have been 'mad' or, in more modern terminology, to have suffered from a manic-depressive psychosis, George is now considered by many physicians to have been a victim of porphyria. Macalpine and Hunter, by a piece of brilliant detective research, traced the disease back through George I's mother, Elizabeth of Bohemia, to her father, James I, and to his mother, Mary Queen of Scots. They then traced the story forward and showed the disease in Queen Anne, great-granddaughter of James I and the last Stuart sovereign, in Frederick I of Prussia, grandson of Elizabeth of Bohemia, in four of George III's sons, and in two living persons, one descended from Frederick I and the other from a sister of George III.

George III, born in 1738 and dying in 1820, had eight attacks of illness, all of a similar character, between 1762, when he was twenty-four years old, and 1804. In October 1810 he again fell ill and, after two years of exacerbations and remissions, lapsed into hopeless insanity; he died, mad, blind and stone deaf at the age of eighty-one. Many attempts have been made to link his 'madness' with the most notable event of his reign, the loss of the American colonies and the birth of the independent United States of America. Undoubtedly George was a stubborn, not very intelligent, unimaginative man and he backed his prime minister, Lord North, in the foolish provocation which precipitated the War of Independence in 1775. But he showed no sign of mental aberration between attacks; he was garrulous, asked strange questions such as 'How does the apple get into the dumpling?', often seemed more interested in turnips than in statecraft; but he ruled adequately and, indeed, with some firmness. He had his second attack, not a severe one, in January-February 1766 and was then free from symptoms until July 1788. The latter was the first major incident, when his mind became so deranged that the House of Commons passed a Regency Bill in January 1789. But, while the Bill was under debate in the House of Lords, the King began to recover. By 10 March he had 'resumed personal exercise of His Royal Authority'. Since there is no evidence of 'madness' between 1766 and 1788 we can hardly hold porphyria to blame for the loss of the American colonies in 1775-6. The King's bad judgement may have precipitated the crisis and his obstinacy may have prevented an amicable settlement, but that bad judgement and that obstinacy were shared by his ministers, the majority of the House of Commons, and a large proportion of the British public.

During the eighteenth century, Protestant settler and Catholic native lived fairly amicably together in Ireland, although Catholics were not allowed to sit in the Dublin Parliament. In the last years of the century, republican France offered to liberate Ireland from the yoke of England, an offer which provoked the rebellion of 1798 when Catholics attempted to set up a Celtic Republic dominated by priests. After the revolt had been cruelly suppressed by a combination of British troops and Irish Protestants, the prime minister, William Pitt, decided that union of the two islands in one Parliament at Westminster offered the best hope of restoring order and justice. He induced the Dublin Parliament to abolish itself and to declare for union with Britain in 1800, on the understanding that Catholics would be eligible to sit in the new United Parliament; in other words, Pitt committed himself to Catholic emancipation.

But he omitted to inform George III of his intention. George regarded himself as the defender of the true Protestant Faith. When the Lord Chancellor drew his attention to Pitt's proposal, the King at once objected and Pitt resigned. Ten days later, in February 1801, George suffered another attack of porphyria with severe mental derangement. When he recovered in March, Pitt gave him his solemn promise that Catholic emancipation would never again be mentioned in the King's lifetime. 'Now my mind will be at ease,' George answered. Thus, in order to set the Royal mind temporarily at rest, the subject of Catholic emancipation was shelved for another twenty-eight years. Lacking this essential ingredient, Pitt's scheme for the pacification of Ireland failed; to the Irish Catholic, union with Britain denoted no more than domination by the alien and oppressive Protestant. Hence developed the troubles of the nineteenth and twentieth centuries.

The genetic disease haemophilia A is transmitted via the female X chromosome. There is a gene borne upon the male X chromosome which will counteract the effect of the female haemophiliac gene if that happens to be present. But there is no room for this counteracting gene upon the small Y chromosome. Thus, when a daughter is born, she will inherit one X from her mother and one X from her father; the gene for haemophilia and the counteracting gene will cancel each other out and she will show no sign of the disease. But the daughter can still *transmit* the disease to the next generation, for the gene is present upon one of her X chromosomes. When a son is born, he may suffer from the disease, since he will inherit either a haemophiliac X or a normal X from his mother but not both, and can only inherit the useless Y from his father. Again, since the haemophiliac gene is upon the X, a haemophiliac father cannot transmit haemophilia to his son, either as the disease or as a carrier. But he can transmit the haemophiliac gene to his daughters, who will then show no sign of the disease in themselves, but will be carriers. The only conjunction which can produce the overt disease haemophilia in a girl is when a haemophiliac man happens to marry a haemophilia-carrying woman. Such an event is unlikely, as it is a rare disease. Haemophilia is nearly always transmitted

174

by the female, who will herself show no sign of the disease, and will appear only in the male offspring.

So Queen Victoria transmitted the sex-linked genetic disease haemophilia first to her daughter Alice and thence to her granddaughter Alix. Alix or, to give her full name, Alice Victoria Helena Louise Beatrice, Princess of Hesse-Darmstadt, was born at Darmstadt on 6 June 1872. At the age of six she lost her young sister and her mother during an epidemic of diphtheria. The family had always visited 'Granny' Victoria once a year; after her daughter's death, the Queen tended to regard the husband as her own son and the visits of the family to the English court became much more frequent.

Alix grew up to be beautiful, a tall slender woman with red-gold hair, blue eyes, a pink and white complexion, her beauty marred only by a withdrawn, cold expression. By no means unintelligent, she had mastered English and German and was well grounded in history, geography, literature and music by the age of fifteen. She also developed a considerable interest in the science of medicine. The great ideals of the Victorian age, hard work, discipline, and service to less fortunate members of society, formed part of the lesson which she remembered throughout her life. She became a prude, the type of Victorian woman who was secretly obsessed by sex but regarded any overt discussion of the subject as disgusting. Not many people knew her well; to those who did, she was 'Sunny', a name given in tribute to her bright hair and sparkling eyes.

In 1884 this quite unimportant princess of a minor royal family travelled for the first time to the court of the mightiest land empire in Europe, the occasion being the marriage of her elder sister to the Grand Duke Serge, brother of Tsar Alexander III. Here she met Alexander's sixteen-year-old son, the Tsarevitch Nicholas, born on 18 May 1868.

If Alix had her genetic problems, so did Nicholas. The root of his trouble lay in that first genetic factor observed by Mendel, the vagaries of tallness. Alexander III was gigantic, six foot six in height, broad in proportion. He could bend a silver coin in his fingers and once held up the roof of a wrecked railway carriage on his shoulders while his family escaped. When the Austrian ambassador tactlessly remarked at the dinner table that it might be necessary to mobilize an army division or two on the frontier, Alexander tied a heavy silver fork into a knot and threw it at him with the words, 'That is what I will do with your divisions'. This great strong bull of a man, downright in word and action, married a tiny woman of more complex character. Nicholas inherited much more from his mother, Maria Dagmar, than he did from his awe-inspiring father. Charming, brave, athletic, shy and hesitant, intelligent, fatally at the mercy of stronger personalities, Nicholas grew into a small man, only five foot six inches tall, surrounded by a mob of gigantic Romanov relations.

The slightly built Nicholas fell deeply in love with the handsome, coldly regal Alix of Hesse, and the match was warmly championed by Queen Victoria, who saw in it a brilliant opportunity for one of her favourite granddaughters. Unfortunately neither Alexander III nor his wife approved, for both of them disliked Germans. Nicholas now showed some of that inner strength and tenacity of purpose which his disastrous reign has tended to obscure. At the beginning of 1892 he told his diary, 'My dream is some day to marry Alix H. I have loved her for a long while, and still deeper and stronger since 1889 when she spent six weeks in St Petersburg. For a long time I resisted my feeling, trying to deceive myself by the impossibility that my dearest dream will come true.' He encountered not only parental opposition. The future Tsaritsa of Russia must be a member of the Orthodox Church. Alix was a fervent Lutheran. Much as she was attracted to Nicholas, this deeply religious, serious-minded girl was not of the type who could regard conversion to an alien Faith lightly.

In February 1894 the forty-nine-year-old Alexander, apparently the strongest and most healthy of men, fell ill of influenza. He may have been already suffering from renal disease, or the attack may have precipitated the trouble. In April he was obviously starting to go downhill and the marriage of the future Tsar quite suddenly became a matter of state importance. Nicholas desired no one else but Alix; there was nothing for his parents to do but to give in.

By October Alexander was desperately ill. Alix, hastily summoned, reached Livadia in the Crimea on 23 October, and the formal ceremony of betrothal took place in the Tsar's bedroom. Typically, the dying man insisted on dressing in full uniform for the occasion. On 28 October comes Alix's interpolation, so prophetic of the future, in Nicholas's diary:

> Sweet child . . . your Sunny is praying for you and the beloved patient. . . . Be firm and make the doctors come alone to you every day—so that you are the first always to know—don't let others be put first and you left out— Show your own mind and don't let others forget who you are.

On 1 November 1894, the mighty Alexander died and the twenty-six-year-old Nicholas II assumed the title of Autocrat, Tsar and Emperor of All the Russias.

Alix's reception into the Orthodox Church under the name of Alexandra Feodorovna, and the marriage on 26 November, took place in an atmosphere of deep mourning. Nicholas, flung into the business of state, could not afford time for a honeymoon. But the prime purpose of a royal marriage, whether a love-match or one of policy, had to be fulfilled; Alexandra did not show herself laggard in her duty. The first child was born in October 1895 and three more followed in the next six years. But each birth proved an increasing disappointment, for in every case Nicholas transmitted an X chromosome and all four were girls. At last, on 12 August 1904, in the middle of the disastrous Russo-Japanese war, the guns of St Petersburg thundered the news of the event which, more than any other, was to change the course of Russian history. That day there was born the unfortunate child Alexis, the longed-for son to whom Alexandra transmitted Victoria's mutant gene of haemophilia.

The first sign of haemophilia showed itself by bleeding from the umbilicus when Alexis was six weeks old; very soon the appearance of bruises, resulting from quite minor knocks while crawling or toddling, confirmed the diagnosis beyond doubt. Alexandra, a devoted mother to all her children, was forced to recognize that she had transmitted the disease to her longed-for son. The revelation came to her as a shock from which she never recovered. No one who has not experienced the bearing of a haemophiliac child can fully understand or enter into the mother's agony. This is why the account written by Mr Robert K. Massie, himself father of a haemophiliac, is a uniquely sympathetic reappraisal of a maligned mother and father.

Of Alexandra Mr Massie writes:

Because she had waited so long and prayed so hard for her son, the revelation that Alexis suffered from haemophilia struck Alexandra with savage force. From that moment, she lived in the particular sunless world reserved for the mothers of haemophiliacs. . . . Haemophilia means great loneliness for a woman. At first, when a haemophiliac boy is born, the characteristic maternal reaction is a vigorous resolve to fight; somehow, somewhere, there must be a specialist who can declare that a mistake has been made, or that a cure is just round the corner. One by one, all the specialists are consulted. One by one, they sadly shake their heads. The particular emotional security that doctors normally provide when confronting illness is gone. The mother realizes that she is alone. Having discovered this and accepted it, she begins to prefer it that way. The normal world, going about its everyday life, seems coldly unfeeling. Since the normal world cannot help and cannot understand, she prefers to cut herself off from it. Her family becomes her refuge. Here, where sadness need not be hidden, there are no questions and no pretensions. This inner world becomes the mother's reality.

Here we have the reason for the parents' withdrawal into seclusion at Tsarskoie Selo, for the bourgeois family life, for the closed and dull confinement to a small court circle; just as Queen Victoria, robbed of her beloved Albert, hid her despair in the suburban castle of Windsor. This kind of existence inevitably bred rumour—that the Tsarevitch could not be allowed in public because of congenital idiocy or epilepsy. And, as the haemophiliac boy was the only direct heir to the throne of Russia, the truth could not be told.

Nicholas could do nothing for Alexis, nor could the doctors or courtiers. The prayers of royal chaplains were equally un-availing and supplications to orthodox saints went unanswered. But God could not entirely desert one who believed in His goodness so fervently, who worshipped Him so wholeheartedly. Somewhere there must exist a human of sufficient spiritual purity and strength to wring from God the miraculous intervention which alone could save the child Alexis. Because such a being was so ardently desired, his appearance was inevitable. It just happened that he took the form of Rasputin, a *staretz* or wandering holy-man.

In July 1907, Alexis lay for three days at the point of death. Rasputin was summoned to Tsarskoie Selo by the Empress, on the advice of either a grand duchess or Alexandra's dowdy but intimate friend, Anna Vyroubova. He sat quietly beside the boy's bed, held his hand, and told him fairy stories and Siberian folk tales. Next day Alexis was free of pain and able to sit up. A temporary 'cure' by this kind of treatment is quite possible; keeping the patient at rest is half the battle.

The next incident falls into a quite different category. In September 1912, when Alexis was eight years old, the imperial family paid a visit to Bialowieza in east Poland. The boy fell when jumping out of a boat and sustained a heavy bruise on the upper part of his left thigh. He complained of severe pain, so the family physician, Dr Eugene Botkin, confined him to bed for a few days. Two weeks later the family moved to Spala, a cramped and dark hunting box in dense forest. Alexis made little progress in these gloomy surroundings, be-came pale and unhappy. Alexandra decided that a long drive would do him good, but the roads were uneven and the carriage jolted unmercifully. After they had gone a few miles,

Alexis started to suffer agonizing pain in his thigh and lower abdomen. Terrified, Alexandra ordered an immediate return. The homeward journey was a nightmare. It soon became obvious that Alexis must be put to bed under medical care as quickly as possible, yet any attempt to speed the horses resulted in increased jolting which caused the boy to scream in pain. By the time they reached Spala he was almost unconscious.

In his fall when jumping out of a boat two weeks earlier, Alexis had fallen heavily on to the butt-end of an oar. The superficial bruising misled the doctors. He had ruptured a small blood vessel, deeply situated in either the upper part of the thigh or the internal abdominal wall. So long as he remained quiet, the bleeding was minimal. The jolting of the carriage not only caused fresh bleeding, but probably widened the rent in the quite small blood vessel which had already been injured.

Nothing would stop the haemorrhage. For eleven days Alexis hovered between life and death, exsanguinated, with a high temperature, tortured by pain. For eleven days Alexandra sat beside his bed, hardly sleeping, snatching brief moments of rest on a sofa in his room. At last the surgeon Fedorov warned the Tsar that his people must be prepared for the heir's death. National prayers were ordered, bulletins were issued, but the nature of the illness was not mentioned. On 10 October priests administered the Last Sacrament, and that day the bulletin was worded in such a manner that the next could announce the death of the Tsarevitch.

That night Alexandra decided to call in Rasputin. He had gone home to Siberia and could only be reached by telegraph. He did not immediately board a train and hurry to Spala. Instead, he telegraphed back: 'God has seen your tears and heard your prayers. Do not grieve. The Little One will not die. Do not permit the doctors to bother him too much.' Twenty-four hours later the bleeding stopped.

There is no doubt that this story is substantially true. Unless the doctors were parties to some mysterious plot, it is also inexplicable. Can we wonder that Rasputin became essential to the mother of Alexis? Is it probable that any report of bad behaviour would turn her against him? Here was the one man for whom she had been praying, a man possessed of the miraculous power to intercede directly and successfully with God. Since God listened to him, Rasputin must be a good man; since he was a good man, anyone who opposed him or spoke evil of him must necessarily be bad. It was as simple as that.

Despite the many books written about Rasputin he still remains a mystery. He was born Grigori Efimovitch, the son of a horse-dealer, in the Siberian village of Pokrovskoie, probably during the 1860s. The name Rasputin, derived from the Russian word for scoundrel, may have been conferred upon him in youth. Practically uneducated, intolerant of discipline, he grew into a very strong young man. At about the age of sixteen he entered a monastery, but found no satisfaction in a monkish life and returned to Pokrovskoie where he found work as a wagoner. In 1891 he was sentenced to a flogging and a term of gaol at Tobolsk for being accessory to a theft of furs.

From the age of sixteen onwards he acquired the reputation of a womanizer. Rasputin had a singular fascination; very few women could resist him, although he treated them brutally. At about the age of nineteen, he married Praskovie Fedorovna Dubrovin, a girl from the neighbouring village. She bore him a son who died when aged six months, and Rasputin quite suddenly became deeply religious. He set out to walk 2,000 miles to the monasteries of Mount Athos in Greece and then decided to trudge on to the Holy Land. Two years later he returned to Pokrovskoie, a changed man. He travelled about the countryside preaching, and gained a wide local reputation as a holy man who had the gift of prophecy and could cure illness by the laying on of hands. He also became noted for generosity; when his admirers made him gifts, he usually passed them on to more needy people. From time to time he returned to Pokrovskoie, where his wife bore him three more children. He was a loving husband and father but entirely unfaithful. He even seduced women who came to hear him preach.

This sort of life continued for about ten years, while his reputation for saintliness steadily grew and spread. In 1903 he seems to have been in Kiev and is said to have encountered the Grand Duchess Anastasia, one of the daughters of King Nikita of Montenegro, who was married to the Grand Duke Nicholas Nicholaievitch, a cousin of Alexander III. Anastasia invited Rasputin to visit St Petersburg where, during a stay of five months, he established friendly relations with many of the leading clergy including Alexandra's confessor, Father John Sergieff of Cronstadt.

Rasputin left the capital to resume his wandering, preaching life, but returned to St Petersburg early in 1905. At first he shared a flat with several other people and lived quietly, gaining a reputation for holiness and an ability to cure sickness. The latter power brought him into contact with Grand Duke Nicholas. Nicholas had a pet dog to which he was devoted. When the dog fell ill Nicholas, presumably on his wife's advice, called Rasputin in, and was very impressed by his treatment. There is nothing magical about this; obviously Rasputin, the son of a Siberian horse dealer, had a working knowledge of veterinary medicine. But from Nicholas it was only one step to the Tsar, and Rasputin had already gained the friendship of clergy who entered the royal circle. Thus, on 1 November 1905, the Tsar recorded in his diary, 'We have today met a man of God, Gregory, from the province of Tobolsk.'

How well Rasputin merited Nicholas's description 'a man of God' is open to question. It is difficult, but not impossible, to combine piety with lechery. He probably was a sincerely pious man. One theory proposes that he fell into an ancient heresy which held that, because Christ came to save sinners, no man can enter into salvation unless he first sins. Another suggests that Rasputin adhered to the Khlysty sect, deviants from the Orthodox Church, whose practices were erotic and deeply rooted in paganism. During the first years in St Petersburg he was something of an ascetic, a vegetarian who rarely touched alcohol. Not until about 1910 did his wild drunken orgies become notorious. As one of the few people who gained admission to the closed circle of Tsarskoie Selo, Rasputin was obviously of use to anyone who desired to influence governmental policy. Rasputin could hardly be expected to choose his entourage wisely, and this is the worst, most disastrous aspect of his hold on the Royal Family.

But, even in the days when he was unknowingly destroying all confidence in the Imperial regime, Rasputin's advice was by no means always bad. He possessed plenty of common sense and he knew his fellow peasants. During the war, he continually urged more equitable division of food supplies, and he prophesied serious trouble unless something was done to speed up distribution and so prevent long queues waiting for hours in the bitter cold. His prophecy proved correct, for the revolution started in the food queues of Petrograd. Had the empress been less dependent upon him, his presence at court could have been a stabilizing influence, for the majority of peasants were less impressed by stories of his orgies than by the fact that one of their number had broken through the barrier of the nobles to reach their Little Father the Tsar.

Great saint or great sinner? Rasputin was something of both. The same kind of question must be asked of his ability to arrest the internal bleeding which caused Alexis agonizing pain and jeopardized his life. Was he in league with the royal physicians who told him the exact moment at which to exercise his alleged power? Did he have access to 'mysterious Tibetan remedies' supplied by the quack doctor Peter Badmaiev? Was it done by hypnosis? Had he stumbled on the possibility that all disease, even uncontrollable haemorrhage itself, may be psychosomatic and that cure can be aided by psychiatric treatment? Or was it just luck? We shall never know the answer to this question, but the essential fact is that Alexandra firmly believed in Rasputin's power.

There is evidence that the Tsar did not altogether share his wife's obsession. Nowhere in his diary, in his letters to his mother or to Alexandra, does he so much as mention the miraculous power of Rasputin. He attributed the recovery at Spala to administration of the Last Sacrament. Nicholas regarded Rasputin as an ordinary Russian peasant: 'He is just a good, religious simple-minded Russian. When in trouble or assailed by doubts, I like to have a talk with him, and invariably feel at peace afterwards.' The Tsar, who received the police reports, must have known much better than did Alexandra of Rasputin's scandalous life, and he was probably at times disturbed by her dependence upon one who, however good and simple, behaved in so dissolute a fashion. There is a story that a courtier, Admiral Nilov, asked the Tsar why he continued to put up with Rasputin's insolent behaviour. 'Better Rasputin than hysterics,' answered Nicholas shortly.

The scandal of Rasputin did not become an urgent problem until the First World War. 'Holy fools', soothsayers and monstrosities had always formed part of the Russian court retinue. Rasputin was not the first wonder-worker to gain access to Tsarskoie Selo: Alexandra had at one time been so influenced by a charlatan named Philippe Nizier-Vachot that she had developed a pseudocyesis or false pregnancy. And there is no evidence that Rasputin exerted real political influence before August 1915, although he sometimes backed private petitions with his name. He rarely visited the imperial family, probably not more than half a dozen times in any one year. But his association with Tsarskoie Selo, his intimacy with some of the grand duchesses, wealthy industrialists and wives of the nobility, his public drunkenness and notorious lechery, were reported in the press (then uncensored) and alarmed many responsible Russian leaders.

In July 1914, when war became imminent, Rasputin was at home in Siberia, convalescing from a stab wound. When he heard of the order for mobilization, Rasputin telegraphed to Tsarskoie Selo: 'Let Papa not plan war for with war will come the end of Russia and yourselves and you will lose to the last man.' The Tsar angrily tore the telegram in pieces. He wished to take immediate command of his beloved army and was only with great difficulty persuaded to appoint as commander-in-chief the Grand Duke Nicholas Nicholaievitch, the most experienced soldier in the imperial family. The war went badly for Russia: the Battle of Tannenberg on 26-30 August saved France by diverting German troops from the western front but almost destroyed the regular army. Lack of munitions continually hampered recovery; although Russia achieved some startling successes against Austria, she could make no headway against Germany. By August 1915 nearly 4 million men had been lost and so had most of Poland. At this critical time the Tsar decided to take command. He did so against the advice of all his ministers, but with the enthusiastic support of Alexandra.

Alexandra's eagerness for this absurd, although understandable, move on the Tsar's part was dictated by her determination that her husband must never be second to anyone in the Empire. On 24 June 1915, she wrote to Nicholas, then touring the front lines:

Sweetheart needs pushing always and to be reminded that he is the Emperor and can do whatsoever pleases him—you never profit of this—you must show you have a way and will of yr. own, and are not led by N [Grand Duke Nicholas] and his staff, who direct yr. movements and whose permission you have to ask before going anywhere. No, go alone, without N, by yr. very own self, bring the blessing of yr. presence to them.

From 5 September 1915, when Nicholas left Tsarskoie Selo to take up command of his armies, until 20 March 1917, the day before his arrest at Moghilev, we can follow the tragic and almost incredible events of these last months of tsardom through the letters which passed between Nicholas and his wife. These letters form one of the most astonishing and important of historical documents. But no one can possibly understand them unless he recognizes *and sympathizes with* the terrible dependence of these unfortunate parents upon one who could restore their beloved son to health.

On 4 September, Alexandra had written to the Tsar: 'Do not fear for what remains behind.... Lovy, I am here, don't

laugh at silly old wifey, but she has trousers on unseen.'
Nicholas was overjoyed: 'Think, my wifey, will you not come
to the assistance of your hubby now that he is absent? What a
pity that you have not been fulfilling this duty for a long
time or at least during the war!' On 10 September, Alexandra
accepted her commission: 'Oh Sweetheart, I am so touched
you want my help, I am always ready to do anything for you,
only never liked mixing up without being asked.' Thus, by
these few absurdly childish words, was the supreme government of Russia handed over to the empress. Loving power,
she accepted gladly. But she still demanded to be dominated;
there was only one man upon whom she could now lean, and
that man was Rasputin.

The Tsar started his reign determined to uphold the sacred
principle of autocracy but, in the near revolution of 1905, he
accepted a compromise—a form of parliamentary government
called the Duma. Not so Alexandra, who detested the Duma
for two reasons. First, the Duma instigated public inquiry
into the scandalous behaviour of Rasputin. Secondly, the very
existence of the Duma implied a check upon the absolute
authority of her husband and, worse still, upon the future
autocracy of her son. Her sick fear for the child was translated
into a determination that he must reign as a powerful monarch. To this end, Nicholas must himself be Ivan the
Terrible, Peter the Great, a harsh tyrant who held the unchallenged power in his own hands and could transmit it
intact to his son. Again and again, she returned to this theme
in her letters: 'For Baby's sake we must be firm as otherwise
his inheritance will be awful, as with his character he won't
bow down to others but be his own master.' 'We must give a
strong country to Baby, and dare not be weak for his sake,
else he will have a yet harder reign, setting our faults to right
and drawing the reins in tightly which you have let loose....
he has a strong will and mind of his own, don't let things slip
through yr. fingers and make him have to build up all again.'
This was the driving force which steered Nicholas into the
fatal errors of the last eighteen months.

Alexandra had no thought of anything, of the country's good, of the war effort; the only criterion was an individual minister's reaction to Rasputin. Her ministers were 'good' if they consulted Rasputin and accepted his advice. At first they were 'bad' only if they actively opposed him but, in the end, they were bad if they neglected to seek his counsel.

On 2 February 1916, the aged Goremykin was suddenly dismissed, to be replaced as premier by B. V. Stürmer, a Master of Ceremonies at the court. At first Stürmer showed himself to be a strong friend of Rasputin and gained the full confidence of the empress ('such a devoted, honest, sure man'), with the result that he received the additional appointment of Minister of the Interior. The fact that he knew little of his duties and made less attempt to carry them out weighed nothing against his support of Rasputin.

Even had he been capable, Stürmer's Teutonic name must have rendered him suspect; many people, among them the Allied ambassadors, thought that he would urge the Tsar to conclude a separate peace. At the beginning of November members of the Duma launched a bitter attack upon him. Alexandra wrote to Nicholas:

> ...for the quiet of the Duma—Stürmer ought to say he is ill and go for a rest for three weeks—being the red flag for that madhouse, it's better he should disappear for a bit and then in December when they will have cleared out—return again.

Nicholas agreed with his wife's description: 'He, as you say rightly, acts as a red flag not only to the Duma, but to the whole country, alas! I hear this from all sides; nobody believes in him.... Alas! I am afraid that he will have to go altogether.' On 22 November he dismissed Stürmer from both his offices, appointing a very able man, Pokrovsky, to the Foreign Office and the senior of the ministers A. F. Trepov (Transport) to the temporary premiership. Alexandra was not in the least pleased:

> Trepov, I personally do not like and can never have the

same feeling for him as to old Goremykin and Stürmer .... if he does not trust me or our Friend, things will be difficult. I told Stürmer to tell him how to behave about Gregory and to safeguard him always.

Trepov lasted until January 1917, to be replaced by the final Tsarist prime minister, Prince Nicholas Golitzyn, whom Bernard Pares described as 'an honest old gentleman in weak health, who was known to the empress as her deputy-chairman of a charitable committee'. Golitzyn, horror-struck at the proposal, pleaded his infirmities and inexperience, but could not disobey the direct imperial command. He need not have worried, for neither he nor Trepov counted for anything in these last days of tsardom. The empress and Rasputin had found an ideal partner to form a triumvirate in the person of A. D. Protopopov, first acting minister and then the last Tsarist Minister of the Interior.

At first sight Protopopov seems a very sensible choice, for he was a vice-president of the Duma.

But in fact, Protopopov was hopelessly unsuited for the post which he took up on 23 September 1916, after repeated appeals from the empress to the Tsar. To start with, he was probably insane; this is the opinion of many Russians who came into contact with him. Some years before, he had suffered from syphilis and had been treated with 'mysterious Tibetan remedies' by the charlatan Badmaiev, who was a possible source of Rasputin's success with the Tsarevitch, and one of the more unsavoury members of 'the Rasputin gang'. There is little doubt that Protopopov suffered from cerebral syphilis; he would probably have died horribly had he not had the good fortune to be shot by the Bolsheviks. He knew nothing of his work, but spent most of his time as Minister of the Interior in drawing up fantastic plans, illustrated with complicated graphs and charts, for sweeping reforms of the army, the government and the whole nation. He rarely troubled to attend meetings of the cabinet or Duma.

Nicholas doubted the wisdom of retaining a madman as one of his most important ministers:

I am sorry for Prot.—he is a good, honest man, but he jumps from one idea to another and cannot make up his mind on anything. I noticed that from the beginning. They say that a few years ago he was not quite normal after a certain illness (when he sought the advice of Badmaiev). It is risky to leave the Ministry of Internal Affairs in the hands of such a man in these times.... Only, I beg of you, do not drag our Friend into this. The responsibility is with me, and therefore I wish to be free in my choice.

Unfortunately for Russia, Rasputin and Alexandra were determined that Protopopov should not go. The Tsaritsa delivered one of her heaviest broadsides on her unfortunate husband:

I entreat you don't go and change Protopopov now—he is all right—he is honestly for us. Oh, Lovy, you can trust me. I may not be clever enough—but I have a strong feeling and that helps more than the brain often. Don't change anybody until we meet, I entreat you, let's speak it over quietly together ... Protopopov venerates our Friend and will be blessed ... He is *not* mad, the wife sees Badmaiev for her nerves only.... Quieten me, promise, forgive, but it's for you and Baby I fight.

Two days after sending this letter, Alexandra set out for the Tsar's headquarters and stayed there for three weeks. It was not an easy visit, for Nicholas proved unexpectedly obdurate. He argued that there was antipathy to Protopopov on every side; she pleaded with him to be firm, to be 'sharp and bitter', to show that he was the master who took no account of popular clamour. Above all, he must trust in Rasputin. 'Ah, Lovy,' she had written, 'I pray so hard to God to make you feel and realize that He is our caring; were He not here, I don't know what might have happened. He saves us by his prayers and wise counsels and is our rock of faith and help.' On the day that Alexandra left him, Nicholas wrote apologizing for having been so 'moody and un-restrained'. But she had got her way. Protopopov was confirmed in his office, to guide the empress and Russia to their downfall with the help of Rasputin.

The Tsar, his wife and Rasputin were now, in 1916, intensely unpopular among all classes in Russia. This hatred had developed in a little less than eighteen months. Many well-meaning attempts were made to open the Tsar's eyes to the true position. His own mother, several grand dukes, the British and French ambassadors, the president of the Duma, all warned him of his danger, besought him to get rid of Rasputin and to 'throw in his lot with the people'. Grand Duke Paul, Alexandra's favourite uncle by marriage, and her own sister, Grand Duchess Elizabeth, pleaded with her to rid herself of Rasputin's influence. They all failed; and as a result, the imperial family decided upon direct action.

According to Bernard Pares, they rather naïvely reasoned that Alexandra would be in a mental home within a fortnight of Rasputin's death and that Nicholas could then be easily persuaded to become a good constitutional sovereign. The young Prince Felix Yusupov, nephew by marriage of the Tsar, instigated the plot, in which he was joined by V. M. Purishkevitch, an ardent monarchist and extreme right-wing member of the Duma, and by Grand Duke Dmitri, the Tsar's favourite cousin and son of the Grand Duke Paul.

At midnight on 29 December 1916, Rasputin visited Yusupov by appointment at his luxurious house in Petrograd. Here had been arranged in a downstairs room some plates of small cakes and decanters of Rasputin's favourite madeira, all well laced with cyanide of potash. Rasputin ate two cakes and drank several glasses of the wine. He then asked Yusupov to play on the balalaika. He sat listening with a drooping head but did not collapse. The other assassins were waiting in a room above; Yusupov excused himself, went upstairs to borrow Dmitri's revolver, and returned. He found Rasputin still sitting with bowed head, breathing heavily. Yusupov shot him in the region of the heart and went upstairs again to announce Rasputin's death. But Rasputin was not dead; he followed Yusupov upstairs, pushed against an outer door and staggered into the courtyard, roaring with fury. Purishkevitch hurried after, fired two shots and missed, fired twice more, and Rasputin fell face downwards in the snow. They hauled him into a car, drove to a bridge over the Neva, and thrust him through a hole in the ice. But even now Rasputin was not dead for, after divers had recovered the body on 1 January, a post-morten examination revealed that the lungs were full of water.

The fact that Rasputin survived the shots is perhaps explicable by his murderers' bad aim due to emotional disturbance. At first sight it is less easy to account for his resistance to the poison. The suggestion usually made is that there never was any cyanide in the cakes or wine—the doctor who provided it had tried to cover himself in the event of the plot's failure by substituting a harmless chemical. There is, however, another and more likely theory. Cyanide kills very quickly when taken orally because it is broken down by the hydrochloric acid normally present in the stomach, to form lethal hydrocyanic acid. A few people have no free hydrochloric acid in the stomach, and this condition 'achlorhydria' is more common among chronic alcoholics. Thus Rasputin, a known drunkard, may quite possibly have survived a large dose of potassium cyanide.

The effect of Rasputin's death upon Alexandra was exactly the reverse of that expected. So far from relapsing into hopeless mania, she completely recovered after the initial shock. One of the most remarkable aspects of the story is the amazing fortitude of this sick woman, who supported the whole family throughout the misery and indignities of the next eighteen months.

The Tsar was the one actor in this drama who totally collapsed. All who met him during the two months between Rasputin's death and his fall from power were startled by his changed appearance and manner. The old charm had gone; his face became lined and apathetic, his eyes lack-lustre and yellowed; he was moody, hesitant, sometimes seeming neither to know the day of the week nor to be aware of his surroundings. Many thought that he drank heavily or took drugs. There is no evidence in support of either supposition, but we can find both a psychological and a physical reason. During the past eighteen months, the Tsar had not only lived under intense strain, but had become completely isolated; all his advisers and his old devoted friends had either resigned in disgust or been removed by order of Alexandra. He must have known that this isolation resulted from his loyalty to his wife and her concept of Rasputin; Rasputin was essential to her and must therefore be retained at all costs. Now Rasputin was gone and his wife seemed almost unmoved; all these sacrifices and mistaken decisions had been unnecessary.

The physical reason is to be found in two of his letters. On 12 June 1915, he wrote in reply to Alexandra's inquiry:

Yes, my darling, I am beginning to feel my old heart. The first time it was in August of last year, after the Samsonov catastrophe, and again now—it feels so heavy in the left side when I breathe.

On 11 March 1917, there is a more ominous paragraph:

This morning during the service, I felt an excruciating pain in the chest, which lasted for a quarter of an hour. I could hardly stand the service out, and my forehead was covered with drops of perspiration. I cannot understand what it could have been, because I had no palpitation of the heart; but later it disappeared, vanishing suddenly when I knelt before the image of the Holy Virgin. If this occurs again I shall tell Feodorov.

The Tsar appears to have suffered from a small coronary infarct or, perhaps, from angina.

Nicholas, although commander-in-chief of the Russian armies, remained at Tsarskoie Selo for two months after the murder of Rasputin. Then General Alexiev summoned him urgently to headquarters, probably because the discipline of some units gave cause for alarm. Olga and Alexis developed measles the day after he left, to be followed shortly by the three other girls and Anna Vyroubova. Alexandra nursed them all devotedly and had little time to spend on the business of government. Protopopov ruled almost alone, with the occasional ghostly advice of Rasputin conjured up in spiritualistic séances.

On the very day, Thursday 8 March, that Nicholas left Tsarskoie, disorders broke out in Petrograd. For the past month the weather had been unusually severe, even for a Russian winter; the railways were brought almost to a standstill and little food or coal could reach the city. There is said to have been plenty of flour but no fuel to bake bread. The Duma furiously attacked the government's food policy, while large crowds wandered aimlessly about the streets, demanding bread, but doing little damage and quietly breaking up when called upon by the police. Next day the crowds increased and many food shops were looted; Cossacks helped the police to restore order, but neither side seemed eager to attack the other.

It was not until Saturday 10 March that any political flavour appeared in the demonstrations. A few of the crowd carried red flags and there were some shouts of, 'Down with the German woman'; in other respects the disorder was no more than a rather widespread food riot. On Sunday, police and troops fired on the crowds. The Pavlovsky regiment mutinied but were disarmed by the famous Preobrazhensky Guards. Order had been entirely restored by nightfall. But, in the course of Sunday's rioting, the Volynsky regiment, which had taken part in the shooting, returned to their barracks in disgust. During the night they mutinied and killed an officer. On Monday morning, 12 March, the Volynsky joined the crowds on the streets. This was the action which changed an aimless bread-riot into a revolution.

Early on Monday morning, the leaders of all left-wing Duma groups met in the flat of Alexander Kerensky and decided that the chance to overthrow the regime, if it had ever existed, had now passed. Three hours later Alexander Kerensky, who later became prime minister of the Provisional

Government, heard of the Volynsky mutiny; he immediately telephoned a friend and instructed him to advise the regiment to go straight to the Duma. The Volynsky accepted this advice and sent deputations to other regiments inviting them to leave their barracks and join them 'in defence of the Duma'. By the evening, the whole of the Petrograd garrison, except for three companies of the Ismailovsky regiment and three companies of Chasseurs, had gone over. The Duma, seeing which way events were moving, refused to dissolve.

But the Tsar was still Tsar, and urgent messages passed between the Duma and headquarters. Late in the evening Nicholas understood that the position had become extremely serious; at 3 a.m. on the morning of Tuesday 13 March, he ordered General Ivanov to Petrograd and himself set out in the imperial train. Ivanov managed to reach Tsarskoie Selo, where he learned that the cabinet had been arrested by the Duma and order restored in Petrograd; he decided there was no point in continuing his journey and returned to headquarters. Nicholas made the fatal mistake of not following Ivanov's train; instead he went south by a branch line which joined the main Moscow-Petrograd railway. When half-way between the junction and Petrograd, his escort received warning that the line was held by revolutionaries and it would be dangerous to proceed. They decided to turn back west in the direction of Pskov where General Ruzsky, commanding the northern front, might be able to deal with the situation. The Tsar reached Pskov on the evening of 14 March.

No one now governed in Petrograd. The Duma had become the centre of a kind of mob rule, feebly trying to restore some semblance of order with the alternate aid and opposition of the Council or Soviet of Workers and Soldiers, hastily elected by show of hands on the basis of one representative per 1,000. During the night of 14-15 March, a prolonged and often angry series of discussions took place between Duma and Soviet; at length they reached agreement that the tsardom should be retained, but that Nicholas must abdicate and Alexis ascend the throne as a constitutional monarch under the tutelage of the Duma and the regency of his uncle, Grand

Duke Michael. Two members of the Duma, the liberal Alexander Guchkov and the monarchist Basil Shulgin, drew up a deed of abdication and left for Pskov at dawn on 15 March.

Meanwhile the generals commanding all the fronts had been busily telephoning one another. They unanimously agreed that the situation could only be saved by the Tsar's abdication. Ruzsky communicated their opinion to Nicholas, who, after some hesitation, consented. At 3 p.m. on 15 March he drew up his own Act of Abdication, naming Alexis as his successor with Grand Duke Michael as regent. He intended that this decision should be telephoned to Rodzianko, as President of the Duma, but Ruzsky learned that Guchkov and Shulgin were on their way to Pskov and advised Nicholas to wait until they arrived.

In the interval of waiting for the Duma representatives, the Tsar changed his mind. He sent for the surgeon Feodorov and demanded to be told truthfully whether his son's illness was curable or incurable. Feodorov replied honestly: medical science knew no cure for haemophilia. When Guchkov and Shulgin arrived at ten o'clock on the night of 15 March, Nicholas told them that he could not be parted from his ailing son. He would abdicate, but only in favour of his brother Grand Duke Michael.

The Duma representatives were horrified, for the whole plan had been wrecked. A boy of twelve under the tutelage of the Duma might have been acceptable; Michael, once banished from Russia and by no means popular, would be just another Romanov autocrat. And so it turned out, for when the deputies proclaimed Tsar Michael at Petrograd station, they were howled down and had difficulty in escaping from the angry mob. Twenty-four hours later Michael, too, abdicated the crown of Russia. Haemophilia had destroyed the last chance of saving the Romanov dynasty.

Would it have made any difference if Nicholas had abdicated in favour of Alexis? Both the Duma and Soviet seem at the time to have been willing to accept him. A young, helpless boy might have inspired sympathy, might have formed a rallying point and allowed the shaken Russian people to regain equilibrium. Morale at the rear, especially in the capital, had reached a very low point, but that morale had collapsed only during the idiocies of the last eighteen months. Morale at the front was surprisingly high; nothing remotely resembling a breakdown occurred until after the March revolution. Adequate supplies of munitions were at last beginning to pour in from Russia's own factories and from Britain. America was on the brink of war with Germany. Both Ludendorff and Hindenburg have written of their anxiety during the summer and autumn campaigns of 1916 on the Russian front. Austria, more exhausted than Russia, had already made peace overtures and was to renew them in 1917. Russia might conceivably have rallied around her young Tsar; then the history of the world would have been very different.

After a summer of anarchy, disillusion, and defeat, the only call which would rally the despairing people of Russia in the autumn of 1917 was that of bread and land and peace. These the minority Bolshevik party promised them and so came to power. In the civil war which followed, the imperial family were taken to the Bolshevik-held town of Ekaterinberg on the eastern side of the Ural Mountains. There, on the night of 16 July 1918, they were all shot by order of the Ekaterinberg Soviet. They died as they had always lived, a united family.

8

Mass Suggestion

Disease can be divided into two types: there is somatic or organic disease, in which the illness depends upon a demonstrable physical lesion; and there is psychiatric disease, in which there is no demonstrable physical lesion. But disease is rarely purely somatic or purely psychiatric. Most somatic illnesses contain a psychiatric element; the very fact that a patient is ill produces symptoms which cannot be related to a definite physical cause. The depression which frequently follows influenza is a simple example. Equally, psychiatric disease often has a physical basis, although that basis cannot be detected by means of a simple medical examination. In some cases the blood chemistry is abnormal, while in others the psychiatrist, when examining his patient, will be able to uncover some physical reason for the disturbance.

Henry VIII suffered from a somatic disease, syphilis, and its effects are apparent in his history. But the effects were exaggerated by his powerful position and by his arrogance and intolerance, which are psychiatric defects. Henry's main trouble was somatic; the psychiatric element was secondary. Napoleon suffered from several minor ills throughout his life, but he thought himself to be a greater man than he was: he conceived for himself the role of a world ruler. In this he was psychiatrically abnormal. His main trouble was psychiatric and his somatic diseases, although they played a large part in his downfall, were secondary.

We find an interesting example of this psycho-somatic combination in the puzzling case of Joan of Arc. From the age of thirteen Joan heard voices and saw visions of saints which commanded her to go to the Dauphin of France, to persuade him to be crowned King, to drive the English and Burgundians from France, and to dedicate his cleansed kingdom to the service of God. In this, Joan was undoubtedly abnormal, for normal people do not hear supernatural voices nor do they see visions. But Joan was certainly not mad; in fact she showed herself thoroughly practical and elaborated a policy which was ultimately successful. It is therefore unwise to dismiss her voices and visions as the hallucinations of a diseased mind; while admitting that she was 'a strange girl', that is, she was psychologically abnormal, we ought to look for a somatic reason for these aberrations of sight and hearing.

The only real evidence is to be found in the evidence which she gave at her trial, and she was very unwilling to speak about her heavenly visitors. Her judges were anxious to show that Joan owed her inspiration to the Black Arts and, at one point, suggested drug addiction. 'What have you done with your mandragora?' they asked. Joan gave a rather curious reply:

I have no mandragora and never had any. I have heard it said that near to my town there is one. I have heard it

said that it is a thing evil and dangerous ... I know not
what use it is.

The mandrake, *Mandragora atropurpurea*, was the source
of the most renowned of mediaeval drugs and was credited
with remarkable powers. It is, however, doubtful whether
mandragora could have produced the type of hallucination
which Joan experienced.

Joan told the court that her Voices first came to her when
she was thirteen years old. When she first heard them, she was
afraid. She could not understand what they said until the
third time, and she could never understand them in noisy
surroundings. Later the figures of saints appeared. She would
give no details of their appearance, but she embraced them
and they had a pleasant odour. Twice she declared that these
apparitions frightened her and she fell on her knees. Then
comes the significant evidence:

I heard the voice on the right hand side . . . and rarely
do I hear it without a brightness. The brightness comes
from the same side as the voice is heard. It is usually a
great light.

Once when she was asleep, the Voice woke her, not by any
touch but by sound alone. The Voice did not seem to be in
the cell where she slept, but was certainly in the castle. She
thanked the Voice by getting up, sitting down on the bed,
and clasping her hands.

A little more evidence is to be found in the Trial of Re-
habilitation, held some years after Joan's death. Two priests
testified that they had visited her in her cell on the morning
of her burning. She told them that her saints (or spirits) came
to her in the form of very minute things, in great numbers
and of the smallest size. The only other suggestive evidence is
the rather mysterious illness which attacked her during her
imprisonment and trial. Her gaolers attributed this to eating
shad—a great Loire delicacy—while Joan blamed a carp sent
to her by the Bishop of Beauvais. Jean Tiphaine, the surgeon

who attended her, wanted more details of her sickness and was told by her attendants that she had vomited on many occasions.

There is insufficient evidence here to make an exact diagnosis, but there is enough to suggest a physical cause. From the age of puberty, Joan suffered from intermittent attacks of severe tinnitus, the annoying singing or ringing in the ears which some patients translate into speech. The tinnitus was unilateral, on the right side only, and was accompanied by visual disturbance which took the form of bright or flashing light mingled with a number of dancing black specks. These specks are, in themselves, a well-known symptom of nausea, which was sometimes so severe that she actually vomited. At the same time she experienced giddiness and was forced to sit down or fall on her knees. She probably suffered from an affection of the right ear, of the semicircular canals which control balance, a type of illness which would nowadays be called Menière's Disease.

But Joan of Arc's somatic disorder is obviously of only secondary importance. She had convinced herself that her Voices demanded the liberation of France. So convinced was she of her mission, that she in turn convinced others and she sparked off a great mass movement. France was in a dreadful state, her people hopeless after seventy years of unsuccessful war and foreign occupation. Joan brought new hope to her countrymen. Here we can put our finger with certainty upon one person who triggered off a great mass-change in behaviour. There are many examples of these mass changes; sometimes we can select the individual who has started the chain reaction; in other cases we can detect no individual stimulus, for there seems to have been a general perception that something which has been accepted without question is undesirable. Such perception will produce mass movements, changes in ways of thought or in patterns of behaviour.

The advance of our civilization may be likened to the imposition of a series of covering skins. Underneath the skins there still lie hidden the primitive instincts of animal Man: fear, hate, anger, greed, self-preservation and preservation of the race. There comes a time in the life of every individual when the skin breaks and the primitive forces its way to the surface. Then the control imposed by civilization is lost; we may rightly speak of the individual's bestial rage or his animal fear. Since men are gregarious, they tend to copy one another and thus, given the right conditions, unreasoning and causeless fear or anger may pass from the individual into the crowd. This is why men or women who are apparently quite sensible in their face-to-face dealings with each other as individuals may, as part of the mass, suffer the delusion, often persistent, that whole categories of their fellow-beings are inimical. There are many instances when one crowd has regarded another, very similar, crowd, as monstrous, as tools of the devil, or as instruments of their own organic decay. This is one of the phenomena usually given the name of Mob or Mass Hysteria.

Mass hysteria in its simplest form is exemplified by the not infrequent occurrence of mass fainting. One girl faints in the workshop, another follows, and a dozen are 'out' within a few minutes. The factory inspector or medical officer holds an investigation. Sometimes he will find a cause; the workshop was unusually hot or the air contaminated by noxious fumes. Quite often, no definite cause is found, but there is probably still a physical explanation. The first girl fainted because she was suffering excessive blood-loss from her period or had come to work without breakfast. The remainder were cases of 'sympathetic fainting'; the fainting was hysterical in that it had no physical cause.

Just as fainting can be contagious, so too can fear, sometimes with tragic results. On 30 May 1883, shortly after the Brooklyn Bridge had been opened, an unreasoning fear that the structure was on the point of collapse swept through the crowd. In the rush to get off the bridge, twelve people were trampled to death and twenty-six seriously injured. The initiating cause of panic is not certainly known. One account states that the bridge began to sway under the weight of the moving crowd, another that someone shouted that the bridge was dangerous, a third that a woman screamed when she fell on a flight of steps. A similar baseless panic caused many deaths on the stairway leading to a deep air-raid shelter during the flying bomb attacks on London in 1944.

Sympathetic fainting and panic fear depend upon mass suggestion, the fainting or panic of an individual suggesting to others that they should follow suit.

The primitive urges of fear, hate, and anger suggest to the individual that he should take immediate and, preferably, violent action. Violent action implies movement, but we cannot always take effectual action; there may be nothing concrete to hit or the object of our protest may be too strong for us. When this demand for action transfers itself from one individual to others a mass movement will result. This may take a bizarre form because the participants cannot translate their protest effectively.

The dancing mania of mediaeval Germany is of particular interest, for here we can find a probable physical cause which initiated the strange behaviour—ergot of rye. One of the chemical compounds found in ergot is D-lysergic acid amide. Lysergic acid diethylamide is commonly known, from its Swiss name Lyserg-Saure-Diethylamid, as LSD. LSD causes hallucinations, agitation, intensely coloured vision, and increases susceptibility to external influences. One of these external influences is rhythm; this is why young people sometimes take the drug before attending pop music sessions. The agitation, hallucinations and heightened perception of rhythm often combine to translate themselves into dancing movements.

Small outbreaks of dancing mania occurred in Germany from early in the Middle Ages until late in the sixteenth century. They were not confined to Germany: the last known 'epidemic dancing' was observed in 1911 close to the Mediterranean outlet of the Dardanelles. The most serious outbreak started at Aix-la-Chapelle in July 1374. It is reasonable to suppose that the initial localized 'epidemic' was due to the eating of rye bread infected with ergot. The sufferers began to dance uncontrollably in the streets, screaming and foaming at the mouth. Some declared they were immersed in a sea of blood, others claimed to have seen the heavens open to reveal Christ enthroned with the Virgin Mary (hallucination).

At first the dancers had no aims, but they rapidly gained adherents who imitated their movements. Thousands were affected and the craze developed into anti-clerical protest. Streams of dancers invaded the Low Countries, moved along the Rhine, and appeared throughout Germany. The cities of Cologne, Mainz and Strasbourg came under a reign of terror. Mobs took possession of monastic houses and shouted abuse at priests, but they did not succeed in dislodging even one of their hated Prince-Bishops. In the later stages, the dancers often appeared to be entirely insensible to pain or other external stimuli, a symptom of hysteria rather than intoxication with LSD. The mania bears a marked resemblance to the flagellant movement which we noticed in Chapter Two. It will be remembered that this started as an intercession against plague and developed into a protest against riches, the Church, and established government.

Both flagellant movement and dancing mania resulted in increased sexual activity. Violent action and violent emotion both stimulate the most primitive instinct, the sexual urge or instinct of race preservation. This stimulation is purposely used as part of the ritual of witchcraft. There is some doubt whether witchcraft is a true return to the primitive. Many people claim to see a remnant of Baal worship and Mithraism; Professor Trevor-Roper argues convincingly that the witch craze was essentially a devil doctrine established by the Church during the Middle Ages. This would certainly account for the marked similarity of witch practices in widely separated countries. There is little evidence that apostles of the diabolical religion travelled widely in search of converts, but there is much to suggest a wide distribution of knowledge through the written and spoken denunciations of churchmen. The mass hysteria of the cult and the hysteria of those who would suppress it are equally interesting. For we cannot divorce the craft from the hunt. If witch hunting took the form of a popular movement at times, then so did witchcraft itself. The cult became widespread at the same periods as did suppression; when we speak of the witch craze, we should not discriminate between the witch and the hunter, but apply the term to both. The three major periods of witch hysteria roughly coincide with the Renaissance, the Protestant Reformation and the Catholic Counter-Reformation. In all three periods we observe a loosening in the hold of conformity which in turn stimulated aberrations and repression. Witchcraft was only one of these aberrations and witch hunting was only part of a general repression of non-conformity, practised by Catholic and Protestant alike.

Much of witchcraft bears the stigmata of hysteria. The myth of the witch on her broomstick flying long distances to the sabbat, is levitation, the sensation of being airborne, and a symptom of hysteria. The sabbat itself with its wild exhausting dance, weird music and sexual orgy is mass hysteria. The feast of nauseous delicacies lacked any taste; the kiss or copulation with a diabolical leader held no warmth. The witch often complained of formication, the sensation that ants were crawling on her skin; the witch finder searched with his bodkin for areas of anaesthesia on the suspect's body —these are well-known symptoms of hysteria.

The witch, endowed with a supposed diabolical power to bring disease and ill-luck, is an object of terror to any man. But we may be able to uncover a more primitive psychopathy among the witch hunters. The witch is usually, though not invariably, a woman who possesses extraordinary powers. She is the embodiment of *feminine* evil. In the celibate priest, in the grim Protestant who believed in the subjection of women, she aroused special hatred and fear. They saw in witchcraft not only an obscene parody of religion but a threat to male supremacy. The witch became a symbol of the primitive love-hate relationship, the age-old struggle for domination between the sexes.

The real increase in witch practices that occurred at the same times as unbridled repression was accompanied by panic exaggeration. Fear bred fear, hatred bred hatred, witches were seen everywhere. The gentle, scholarly Nicolas Remy of Lorraine sent between 2,000 and 3,000 victims to the stake in the years 1595 to 1616. The pious Archbishop of Trier burned 368 witches from twenty-two villages between 1587 and 1593; in two of these villages only one woman remained alive in 1595. From 1623 until 1631 the Prince-Bishop of Würzburg burned 900 people for witchcraft; they included his own nephew, a number of children, and 19 priests. France, Germany, Switzerland, Spain, Sweden, Scotland, all added their quotas of mass murder. Germany was the worst affected, a fact that will have some significance later in this story. At the height of the terror, belief in witches became an article of faith; to deny the existence of witchcraft placed the unbeliever in danger of condemnation.

The worst excesses in England and the American colonies were associated with extreme puritanism, though repression never equalled that on the Continent. Nor, apparently, did witchcraft flourish with the same exuberance. But two outbreaks are notorious. The first affected the eastern counties of England in 1644-7 at a time when the royal cause of Charles I was going down before the puritanical parliamentary armies. The hysterical denunciations and accusations were instigated by Matthew Hopkins, probably a lawyer of Ipswich, who journeyed about the countryside in search of witches. In 1645 he procured a commission as witch-finder general and acquired the judicial support of John Godbolt, a barrister who had been appointed a judge of common pleas for this purpose by vote of parliament. Within just over a year these two villains hanged sixty women in the county of Essex, nearly forty in the town of Bury St Edmunds, and many more in Norwich and Huntingdonshire. Hopkins published a treatise, *The Discovery of Witches*, in 1647, but in the same year was denounced as an impostor by John Gaule, vicar of Great Staughton. Hopkins failed to pass the test of swimming, that is, he floated when thrown into water with hands and feet tied. He was very properly condemned to be hanged as a sorcerer.

The American episode occurred at Salem, then a village about fifteen miles north-east of Boston, Massachusetts. The instigator of this persecution is not certainly known. 'Credit' is usually given to the congregational minister, Cotton Mather, whom we have already met in connection with small-pox inoculation. Mather came of a family of extreme puritans. His grandfather, Richard Mather, emigrated to Boston from Lancashire in 1635. Cotton Mather had a brilliant mind, published nearly 450 books and pamphlets on history, science, biography and theology, was elected Fellow of the Royal Society in 1713, and acquired international fame. He firmly believed in witchcraft and wrote several papers on the subject before 1700, but there is no evidence that he deliberately provoked a hunt. The Salem witch craze began in 1692 with the accusation made by ten young girls that they had been bewitched by two old women and a West Indian slave named Tituba, property of the Reverend Samuel Parris. Parris seems to have been largely responsible for fanning the hysteria, which spread rapidly. Within four months hundreds of women were arrested and tried. The judges condemned nineteen to be hanged and committed many to gaol; one was pressed to death for refusing to plead. There is little doubt that Cotton Mather warned the witch judges that their methods were unfair and that some victims had been unjustly sentenced. The hysteria passed almost as quickly as it had arisen and a swift reaction against the witch hunters followed. In May 1693 Governor Phelps ordered the release of all prisoners held on the charge of witchcraft.

Black magic is the invocation of a malevolent agency to inflict harmful vengeance. It is a labour-saving device: instead of encompassing the harm of an enemy by his own labour, the witch calls upon a supernatural power to do his work. The same is true of white magic, which is essentially similar in the opposite sense: invocation of a benevolent agency to do good. Often it took the form of treating illness; the magic herbs were not efficacious unless gathered with proper ceremonies and swallowed with appropriate incantations. There is here an obvious connection with very old practices, with the Church's ministry of healing which goes back to the dawn of Christianity. But, just as black magic may be the relic of older faiths, so white magic may have its roots in beliefs that are older than the Christian religion. The witch hunters held this opinion, for, in the worst periods of the witch craze, both black and white magic were condemned.

In this the witch hunters were logically correct, for witches, whether black or white, arrogate to themselves powers drawn from a supernatural source. The only difference is that one performs his rites on the whole for evil, the other on the whole for good. The modern teenager who dabbles in black magic is no more atavistic than the Christian Scientist or the priest who credits himself with the ability to heal by intercession and the laying on of hands. In both practices there is a return to the primitive, a regression from reason to superstition. This is not to imply that miraculous cures do not occur. They do. A hysterical person can persuade himself that he is bewitched, and can be equally certain that the spell has been removed. People can deceive themselves that they suffer from the most bizarre complaints. A Wittelsbach princess convinced herself that she had swallowed a grand piano made of glass; Marshal Blücher, one of Wellington's allies at Waterloo, lived in fear of giving birth to an elephant. Many believe themselves to be seriously ill. They are ill because they have persuaded themselves of their illness, although an ordinary medical examination will reveal no sign of disease. Such people can be cured by Christian Scientists, by faith healers, by a visit to Lourdes. They will say that they have been cured by miraculous intervention. They have not. The have been cured by natural means, for their belief in the healing power of the supernatural agency has been sufficient to overcome their own self-deception.

The whole story of Adolf Hitler and the Nazi movement provides a horrible example of what can happen when a diseased individual, a witch hunting craze and mass hysteria are brought together. Hitler himself unwittingly gives us an example of how history may be affected not only by disease itself but by an individual's ideas about disease. Hitler's conception of disease was based upon two assumptions. The first was that society is not merely comparable to a biological organism but that actually and for all purposes it is such an organism. Society is often *compared* to an organism, i.e. 'the body politic', but Hitler, like many before him, mistook the metaphor for reality. In *Mein Kampf* he declared: 'As Aryans, we can consider the state only as the living organism of a people.' His second assumption followed from the first, and is the linchpin of his racist ideology: since human society is a biological organism, it can become diseased or degenerate just as can the individual. Further, just as the union of two individuals may produce a physically or mentally inferior second generation, so the union of two societies or 'races' can result in the degeneration of the product. In order to justify this hypothesis, Hitler had to postulate the existence of a pure stock. So he intensified and developed the 'Aryan myth', the fallacy that Nordic Teutons are pure Aryans. Since he thought that the most immediate threat to Aryan rule and culture came from the supposed 'Jewish race', the Jew was represented as the degenerate element. Hitler's theory of heredity was based on the ancient idea of the literal blending of blood; thus he was able to use such meaningless but provocative expressions as 'poisonous contamination of the race' and 'the pestilential adulteration of the blood'. Logic suggested a further extension of the disease metaphor. Since he regarded the 'Jewish race' as the major contaminant, he depicted the Jew as a bacillus or parasite sapping the vitality of the society in which he lived: 'On putting the probing knife carefully to that kind of abscess, one immediately discovered, like a maggot in a putrescent body, a little Jew who was often blinded by the sudden light.' This concept of *disease* lies at the heart of Hitler's vision of the universe and thus contributed to the most horrifying events in all recorded history. Yet, in a sense, Hitler was right. From 1918 until 1945 he did live in a diseased community. The disease was not physical but of the mind.

In the 1914-18 war Germany made greater sacrifices than any other belligerent. In the spring of 1918 victory seemed to be at last in sight. Russia had signed a humiliating peace treaty at Brest-Litovsk, Rumania had surrendered, the

German armies had at last broken the stalemate of trench warfare and were hurling the Allies back to Paris and the Channel ports. All this was announced to the German people in exultant communiqués. But when the advance faltered, halted, turned to retreat, no inkling of the truth appeared in the press. Knowledge that the military position had become almost hopeless was confined to the High Command. The announcement at the beginning of October that the government was seeking peace terms stunned and bewildered Germany. Up to that moment the home front stood unbroken; the news came as a shattering blow which produced something akin to panic. Even on 11 November, when the government signed the terms of armistice, the armies still preserved their lines on foreign soil and not a single Allied soldier had penetrated German territory.

The economic situation moved from bad to worse. Large numbers of demobilized men, flung on the labour market at a time of high unemployment, added to the general discontent. Demand for reparation payments caused a fall in the mark, from 4 to the dollar in the winter of 1918, to 75 in the summer of 1921, and to more than 7,000 in 1923. The real crisis came in January 1923, when the French government of Raymond Poincaré, convinced that Germany was avoiding reparation payments, moved troops into the industrial district of the Ruhr, thus cutting off 80 per cent of Germany's coal and steel production. By 1 August, the mark had fallen to 1 million to the dollar and to 130,000 million by November. The currency totally collapsed, resulting in loss of all savings, the end of trade, bankrupt businesses, mass unemployment and food shortages in the cities. The foundations of German society were far more shaken by the collapse of the currency than by the war, the revolution of 1918 and the Treaty of Versailles combined.

The world depression, beginning in the USA in 1929 and intensifying during 1930 and 1931, hit Germany particularly severely. In September 1929 unemployment stood at 1,320,000. By January 1932 the figure had reached 6 million. Germany was a sick nation, in that so many of her individual members were mentally sick, defeated and disillusioned, translating their sufferings into a fantasy of persecution.

This was the only Germany that Hitler knew. He had no personal experience of the efficient, prosperous Germany of pre-1914, for he was not a German national. Born on 20 April 1889, at Branau on the frontier between Austria and Bavaria, he was the son of an official in the Hapsburg customs service. His father, Alois, was an illegitimate child of Maria Anna Schicklgruber, the father not being certainly known but presumed to be Johann Georg Hiedler. Alois legitimately adopted the name 'Hitler' twelve years before the birth of Adolf. Although there is no evidence that J. G. Hiedler was a Jew, there is a suggestion that Adolf believed his disputed grandfather to be partly Jewish. Here might be a basis for Hitler's virulent anti-Semitism; there would have been no stigma of illegitimacy in the family tree had his grandmother not been seduced by a Jew. This seems a more likely explanation than the theory, propounded by more than one writer, that he based his obsession upon some sexual experience with a Jewish prostitute.

Adolf Hitler spent his boyhood in a small village outside Linz in Upper Austria. He did badly at school except in such subjects as he, himself, wished to learn; in 1905, aged sixteen, he left without acquiring the customary Leaving Certificate. After his father's death in 1903, he continued to live with his mother. He loved her in his own strange way but did nothing to support the household. Fired with the ambition to become an architect, Adolf made no attempt to acquire a training but spent his time filling notebooks with drawings and elaborate plans for rebuilding Linz. In 1907 he decided to train as an artist in the Academy of Fine Arts at Vienna. He failed the entrance examination and, when he applied again a year later, was not even permitted to retake it. His mother died in December 1907. Adolf, friendless, incompetent and work-shy, disappeared for six years into the slums of Vienna, a world of doss houses, tramps and odd jobs.

But Hitler was more than a mere drop-out. He is an example of that most pathetic being, the would-be creative

artist without talent, training or acquired ability. Of such
are the dreamers who make dreams their master; in their
fantasies the great book is written, the picture painted, the
symphony composed without any intermediate step from
inception to completion. Their dreams never produce anything second-rate; the figment of their minds is always a
masterpiece. So they are themselves great; they find themselves surrounded by a crowd of petty beings who will not
acknowledge their pre-eminence and who hold them down
from their rightful place by jealousy, misunderstanding and
ignorance. Thus the persistent illusion is accompanied by
hatred and contempt of their fellows.

Adolf Hitler's early history clearly shows that he suffered
from paranoia, behaviour dependent upon a fixed belief
totally divorced from reality. He was of the schizophrenic
type which believes itself to be the subject of persecution and
whose actions are dictated by a revulsion against the supposed persecutors. Paranoia caused his indolence, his sudden
bursts of feverish work when work was inescapable, his
maniacal rages when affairs would not arrange themselves
exactly as he wished, his alternating moods of sullen despair
and irrational hope. But how on earth did such a man ever
achieve supreme power?

He would never have done so had it not been for his
service in the First World War. Had it not been for that
service, his sordid career would have ended in gaol, by
suicide or in an asylum. When he was twenty-five war conditions gave him exactly what he needed: inescapable reality,
an outlet for violence, membership of a gang, the security
of discipline. He had evaded compulsory military service before the war, but the moment it broke out he voluntarily
enlisted. Instead of joining the Austrian army, he asked to be
accepted into a Bavarian regiment. Because he offered his
services voluntarily to the army of a country which he
admired and because he found therein the stabilizing conformity which he required, Hitler made a good soldier. He
ended the war a more competent, more stable man than in
1914. But he still suffered from paranoia, was still obsessed

with the delusion that he towered far above his fellow men. He had always been interested in politics, expressing his opinions with an intemperate violence, showing no control in face of debate or reasoned opposition. Such a man has no use for the forms of democratic government. Because *he* was a Teuton, the Aryan élite must be the Master Race. Therefore it was their mission, under his leadership, to restore broken Germany to her former greatness. This Hitler could only do by winning absolute power.

Hitler's party was the party of discontent, of envy, of resentment. The ex-officer like Göring, disappointed intellectuals such as Alfred Rosenberg and Goebbels, out of work labourers, the small shopkeeper ruined by inflation, all these found a place in it. Hitler refused to permit a class or age identification. 'These fine chaps, what sacrifices they were willing to make,' wrote Hitler of his plebeian followers. 'All day at their jobs, and all night off on a mission for the Party. I specially looked for people of dishevelled appearance. A bourgeois in a stiff collar would have bitched up everything.' The bourgeoisie had failed to support Hitler, had forced him to scratch a living in the gutters of Vienna; although he had to have their support for, unlike Lenin, Hitler could not ride to power on the shoulders of the workers alone, he felt nothing for them but contempt.

During the thirteen years of Hitler's struggle towards power, his organization reached its tentacles into the heart of German youth. Hitler Youth, that frightful parody of scouting, was founded about 1926 and grew quickly in strength; six years later over 100,000 members paraded before their Leader in the torch-lit stadium at Potsdam. The Students' League and the Nazi Schoolchildren's League were other methods of indoctrination. The active spearhead of Nazism, the S.A., rose rapidly in numbers, from 27,000 in 1925 to 178,000 in 1929. But Nazism, the party of discontent, could make little headway when Germany was struggling back to prosperity in the years 1923-9. Hitler's turning point came with the economic depression. In 1928 the Nazis polled 810,000 votes at the Reichstag elections; in 1930 they polled

6,409,600, about a fifth of the total cast, and in 1932 they gained no less than 13,745,000. Hitler had now become a political force. More ominous was his turbulent S.A., which he himself found difficulty in controlling. Drawn largely from the ranks of the unemployed, they now numbered over 400,000, four times the size of the regular army permitted by the Treaty of Versailles.

Adolf Hitler came to power on 30 January 1933. He commanded only 37 per cent of the national vote, and he achieved his ambition not by a great upsurge of patriotic heroism (as the carefully fostered legend declared), but by a shoddy deal with the parties of the Right, the 'Old Guard' whom he and his followers had been attacking for years past. The Right aimed to regain its old function as the ruling class, to destroy the Republic and to restore the Hohenzollern monarchy, to repress the workers and their trades unions, to reverse the Treaty of Versailles and to rebuild the military power of Germany. Led by the octogenarian Hindenburg, now in his dotage, and by the aristocratic Franz von Papen, they made the fatal mistake of believing that in Hitler they had found the man to help them attain their ends. They put their trust in Hitler's good intentions and in the promises which he made. They were not alone. Neville Chamberlain and Edouard Daladier among others fell into a similar error. Psychiatry is not a compulsory subject in the training of politicians, so we cannot altogether blame them if they failed to understand that a paranoiac does not behave in a rational manner.

So Germany passed into the rule of the gang. The gang demanded conformity with its laws and usages. Nazism, purged of its radical element at the end of June 1934, became the only political party in Germany, with Hitler as its leader and dictator of policy. There followed a witch hunt, the extermination of every person who would not conform to the pattern of the gang. Since Hitler had declared that Jews were the diabolical agents or instruments of organic decay, the Jewish race necessarily suffered the greatest hardship. They were persecuted, just as witches had been persecuted in sixteenth- and seventeenth-century Germany, but with all the refinements made possible by technological advance. Some 9 million people died in German-controlled concentration camps during the years 1934-45, and 6 million of them were Jews. To the earnest Nazi, the Jew was an animal, a non-man; the Nazi had reverted to the thinking of his remote ancestors who described themselves as 'the men', thus implying that other tribes, groups, or villages had no part in human virtues or in human nature.

The Nazis desired to preserve that race and they feared and hated anything which menaced their self-preservation. Thus the primitive instincts of fear and hate, self-preservation and race-preservation broke through the skins of civilization and came to the surface. The despairing Germans of the 1920s and early 1930s deliberately sloughed off those thin skins or veneers under which Primitive Man lies hidden. They found their immediate satisfaction in violence, conformity and the gang. The whole Hitler episode—with its hysterical Nuremberg rallies, indoctrinated youth, witch-hunts, and insane racial theories—was a return to the hates and lusts and fears of Primitive Man. It is a terrible example of the dangers of mass suggestion.

9
Man-made Problems
of the Present and
Future

There is a term 'iatrogenic conditions' which is being increasingly used by doctors. It implies illnesses or disabilities that can be attributed to the physician's treatment. This is a measure of the complexity of modern medicine. A drug may be invaluable in the cure of a certain disease, yet have distinct and sometimes dangerous disadvantages. The outstanding example is *thalidomide*, which appeared to be a very great advance. When introduced in 1956, it was hailed by the lay press as 'a major break-through'. Thalidomide lacked the dangerous drawbacks of the barbiturate group of drugs which are commonly used to induce sleep. It appeared to be non-habit-forming and to possess so wide a margin of safety that overdose was impossible; only the would-be suicide disapproved of thalidomide. So safe that it could be sold across the counter without prescription and could be given to very young children, it became known as 'the West German babysitter'.

In 1959-61 West German paediatricians found themselves being consulted about a very unusually high number of children suffering from the deformities known as phocomelia or 'seal extremities', a rare congenital deficiency of the long bones which produces normal or rudimentary hands and feet springing directly from the trunk. These unfortunate children also suffered from deformities of the eyes, ears, heart, alimentary and urinary tracts. In ten West German clinics no case had been seen for ten years prior to 1959. In 1959 these ten clinics experienced 17, in 1960 126, and in 1961 no less than 477 cases. This remarkable increase seemed at the time to be confined to Germany. Most doctors considered that there had been an unobserved surge in radioactive fall-out or that the mothers had been exposed to overdoses of Roentgen rays. The mothers were questioned very closely. One doctor, W. Lenz of Hamburg, asked them to list all the drugs that they had taken during pregnancy. On examining the results he found that 20 per cent of the mothers had taken a mild, harmless sedative and hypnotic drug called Contergan.

Dr Lenz found that Contergan was the drug most frequently mentioned and decided to re-question his group. Now, almost exactly half of the mothers of affected children admitted having taken Contergan in early pregnancy; most of them said they had not troubled to mention it before because it was such a harmless drug. On 20 November 1961, Lenz attended a meeting of paediatric physicians at Düsseldorf when thirty-four cases of phocomelia were discussed. He was not yet sure of his facts and had no desire to incriminate a very useful sedative, so contented himself with the suggestion that an unnamed drug, rather than radiation, might be responsible. After the meeting, a physician asked Lenz, 'Will you tell me, confidentially, is the drug Contergan? I ask because we have such a child and my wife took Contergan.' In the next few days Lenz received a number of letters asking the same question.

Meanwhile Dr W. G. McBride of Hurstville, New South Wales, had been consulted about three babies born with phocomelia in April 1961 and about three more born in October and November. On inquiry, he found that all six mothers had taken a mild sedative named Distaval in early pregnancy. In December 1961 he wrote a letter to the *Lancet* asking if similar results of taking Distaval had been reported in England. Lenz replied with his conclusions about Contergan, and reports came in of 17 cases of phocomelia in Birmingham, 33 in Liverpool, and 10 in Stirling. It was later found, on examination of a series of British cases, that no less than 41 of the mothers of 46 affected babies had certainly taken Distaval at some time between the fourth and ninth week of pregnancy, while no case of phocomelia had occurred in the babies of 300 mothers who had certainly not taken Distaval.

Similar cases were reported from many other countries. In the USA this mild sedative was known as Kevadon but experimental trials in 1960 had shown that the drug might have certain undesirable side-effects. Approval for marketing was therefore delayed and had not yet been given when reports of phocomelia started to come in from Europe. But Kevadon had already been given to 1,270 doctors for clinical trial; it is reckoned that these doctors distributed it to 20,771 patients, of whom over 200 were pregnant.

Contergan was withdrawn from the German market in November 1961 and Distaval from the British market in December, but cases of phocomelia were still reported. Part of the trouble lay in the number of trade names for thalidomide: Contergan, Distaval, Kevadon, Talimol, Softenon are some. Another reason was that the warnings issued were not sufficiently urgent; bottles of tablets still remained in the family medicine cupboard and continued to be used. Damage to the foetus did not occur unless the drug was taken between the thirty-seventh and fifty-fourth day from the first day of the last menstrual period and, even if taken during this very narrow margin of time, harm was not inevitable. It is reckoned that about 20 per cent of women who took thalidomide during the critical days produced deformed children. The West German Health Ministry estimated that use of the drug resulted in about 10,000 abnormal babies, of whom half survived, 1,600 being so severely affected that they needed artificial limbs. In Britain there were at least 500 cases, of whom some 275 survived. Thalidomide is one of the outstanding examples of something which seemed to meet a public need, to add an amenity to life, to replace a more dangerous agent, yet which carried an unsuspected and more lethal danger. The long-term effects of the contraceptive pill may also cause trouble, such as thrombosis, while it is already well-known that multiple births may result from use of fertility drugs.

A great part of our civilized life depends upon the addition of amenities, the comforts and the pleasures which make a man's existence not only tolerable but happy. Very few of these amenities are entirely innocuous. It is nice to sit beside a fire on a winter's evening, to light our homes with electricity, to drive out into the country in a motor-car on a sunny day. There is no doubt that we are healthier and little doubt that we are more comfortable than our forefathers who lived in cold, dark houses and whose only means of transport was by foot or on horseback. But this does not mean that an open coal fire, electricity and the motor-car are unmixed blessings. All three can cause unnecessary death and all three add to the hazards of city life by polluting the atmosphere.

Atmospheric pollution was an obvious problem in nineteenth-century industrial towns, obvious because no one attempted to clean the products of combustion of their solid content. In such a city as London, built on the marshy plain beside the River Thames and almost encircled by hills, there must have been days of mist even in Roman times. Such mist, composed of water vapour, caused no harm. When 'sea coal' fires came into use in the thirteenth century, the mist was impregnated with dangerous products, chiefly sulphur dioxide, carbon dioxide and solid particles of soot. Pollution increased as the city grew and as factories were built in the environs. Impregnation of the mist with solid particles produced the 'pea-souper' or 'London Particular', the heavily contaminated yellow-brown fog which is the familiar background of the Sherlock Holmes stories and the Charles Dickens novels set in nineteenth-century London. This fog was definitely harmful; it caused a great increase in respiratory diseases, particularly chronic bronchitis. But very heavy pollution at ground level is not common, because the earth is usually warmer than the air above it. The warm air rises and so carries the products of combustion to a higher level. This is why, on a sunny day in the city, visibility may be almost perfect in the streets yet the sun appears to be obscured by haze.

Occasionally the normal pattern is reversed. In prolonged anticyclonic weather conditions and when a city lies in a basin, the upper air may become warmer than that at ground level. There is then no upward flow and the upper, heavily contaminated layer will tend to fall. Such incidents must have occurred in the nineteenth century but they went unnoticed. The first event to draw attention to this problem was in December 1930, when a heavy fog caused an unusual number of deaths in the Meuse valley of Belgium; in October 1948 a similar episode occurred in the city of Donora, USA. Both localities were heavily industrialized; emanations from coke ovens, blast furnaces, and zinc-reduction plants added to contamination from ordinary sources.

The 'smog' incident of London in December 1952 is a little different, for pollution was predominantly caused by domestic coal fires. Pollution started to rise on 5 December and reached its maximum three days later. Analysis of the 'smog' showed that sulphur dioxide content rose to seven times the ordinary figure and that the solids, visible smoke or soot, were no less than ten times the normal. There were a great many deaths, largely among infants and elderly people, and these were due to a rise in mortality from respiratory and cardiac diseases. In the week before the 'smog', 74 people died in Greater London from bronchitis and 206 from coronary disease; in the 'smog week' the figures were 704 and 526 respectively. Thus there were slightly over double the number of deaths from coronary disease and almost ten times the number from bronchitis.

In July 1970 abnormal weather conditions produced ground-level pollution on a very wide scale. The cause was similar, an anticyclone producing a windless atmosphere with temperature inversion. During the week 21-8 July, sulphur dioxide content rose to 0.45 parts per million of air in many cities; the danger level is considered to be 0.10 parts per million. New York seems to have suffered because of the canyon-like streets running between tall buildings and containing an enormous number of petrol-driven vehicles, but power generators added their emanations to the exhaust fumes. Mayor Lindsay warned that it might be necessary to ban automobiles from the city until conditions improved. Tokyo was particularly badly affected and a similar ban was considered. In Tokyo and other Japanese cities factory fumes added greatly to the pollution. Smarting eyes, sore throats, and increased production of phlegm were some of the reported symptoms. Pollution seems also to have caused withering of plants, the sudden death of trees and the disappearance of fish.

Man's pollution of his surroundings is not confined to the air. In June 1969 fish suddenly died in massive numbers along a 250-mile stretch of the River Rhine. The Rhine is known to have a high level of 'normal' pollution from industrial effluents, but this incident could not possibly be regarded as 'normal'. Some 40 million fish, almost the entire population of the 250-mile stretch, died between 19 June and 24 June. An escape of nerve gas was suspected, but, later, Dutch and German authorities agreed that the trouble had occurred because 100 kilogrammes (220 pounds) of the insecticide Endosulfan or Thiodan had accidentally found its way into the Rhine, probably from a barge. Endosulfan is one of the persistent insecticides, remaining active and unchanged in the soil or water for a long time after use.

The Rhine accident is only one episode of a long, continuing tale. Noxious chemicals have escaped from human control on many occasions. In 1968 more than 6,000 sheep died mysteriously in Utah. The United States Army maintained a chemical and biological-warfare testing ground nearby and had inadvertently sprayed an area outside the confines with a nerve gas. The gas drifted for about forty miles before being washed down by a rainstorm. Had it not been for this lucky storm, the gas might have drifted on to a busy highroad in one of the more densely populated parts of Utah. In 1961 a persistent insecticide, DDT, found its way into the Colorado River and killed fish for a 200-mile stretch below Austin, Texas. In 1967 occurred the 'Smarden incident', when leakage of a highly poisonous insecticide from a Kent factory into a small stream and the surrounding soil caused a great destruction of livestock. In 1968 a discharge of cyanide into the Chelmer River, Essex, resulted in the destruction of fish.

These are accidents. Much more revealing is the proud announcement of the Port of London Authority that a live carp had been caught in the River Thames at Fulham, West London, in 1969. Once upon a time, the Thames was a notable salmon river; indeed there is an old legend that London apprentices demanded as one of the articles of indenture that they should not be required to eat salmon more than twice a week. Whitebait and the famous Thames flounder were regularly caught as high up the river as Greenwich, now in Greater London, until early in the nineteenth century. Then the Thames became nothing better than a drain. Sewage and factory effluents poured into the river from the packed city, poisoning the water by removing available oxygen and thus sterilizing it of higher forms of life until only bacteria and mud worms remained. This broadest of the city highways, which must once have been a delight to the eye with its sparkling blue water, green banks, swans, and busy traffic, became a noisome ditch, bordered at low tide with banks of filthy mud. The Victorian gentlemen of the House of Commons sometimes found it necessary to suspend their sittings because the stench offended their not over-sensitive nostrils. Such is the havoc that man can wreak upon his surroundings and, in so doing, endanger his own health and comfort.

The case of the Thames is not unique. Unplanned industrialization has permitted pollution of the air and sterilization of the rivers and countryside. Nor can industry alone be blamed. In the year 1970 Edinburgh, the lovely capital city of Scotland, discharged more than 53 million gallons of untreated sewage into the Firth of Forth every day. Shellfish from the Forth must not be eaten, for they have been found to contain salmonella, shigella, and paratyphoid organisms which cause acute food poisoning, dysentery and enteric fever. A century ago 80,000 salmon were netted from the River Tyne every year. Now most of the effluent from this highly industrialized area together with the untreated sewage from 1 million people is pumped into the river and there is practically no fish life. 'Anyone who falls into the Tyne is liable to die not from drowning but from poisoning,' *The Times* remarked on 23 March 1970.

Nor is the sea inviolate. The spoil from coalmines in Durham and Northumberland is dumped along the beaches and may be washed by tide and current for distances of ten miles. New York's 'Dead Sea' is a twenty-mile-square area twelve miles off the Long Island coast, so heavily polluted by years of sludge-dumping that tide and current cannot wash the noxious material away. In the 1930s a Swedish mining company disposed of 7,000 tons of arsenic by sinking it in the Baltic. The British Ministry of Defence sank 100,000 tons of toxic gases in the Atlantic, Baltic and Irish Seas after the Second World War. In 1970 the United States government disposed of 27,000 tons of nerve gases in one of the deepest parts of the Atlantic. Ships continually discharge unwanted oil and oil residues into the sea; sometimes, as happened in the *Torrey Canyon* shipwreck off the Isles of Scilly, whole tanker-loads of oil are transformed into a vast slick which fouls beaches many miles away.

The artificial manures, pesticides, weedkillers and antibiotics which increase our food supply can also cause trouble. The most important chemical fertilizers are nitrates—those semi-essentials to increased production which food faddists sometimes call 'the devil's dust'. Nitrates are very soluble in water and much of the salt is lost by drainage off the land. This strongly nitrated solution may affect the balance of life in lakes and rivers, causing a large increase or 'bloom' of algae. Excessive algal growth results in disoxygenation of the water, destruction of fish and blocking of purifying machinery. Seepage of nitrates from agricultural land is thought to have been one of the causes of the disastrous alteration in balance of the American Great Lakes. Nitrates are not themselves harmful to adult humans who can drink adulterated water safely, but in young children an enzyme converts the nitrate to nitrite which is highly poisonous. Deaths of babies in America and Europe have been attributed to this cause.

Antibiotics pose a different problem. Battery hens and broiler chicks are very susceptible to infectious disease because they are reared in crowded, confined buildings. Until recently they were fed with foodstuffs treated with antibiotic drugs. The most commonly used was chloramphenicol, which is efficacious against epidemic disease of fowls and against human typhoid fever. Bacteria can develop strains that are resistant to any antibiotic. If the wide use of chloramphenicol produced a resistant strain of typhoid bacillus, the best means of treating the human disease would be useless. 'Routine feeding' of any antibiotic to any farm stock is dangerous for a similar reason; it is therefore essential to exercise strict control of antibiotics.

The persistent insecticide DDT, or Dicophane, was first used to destroy body lice during an outbreak of typhus fever at Naples in December 1943. DDT is lethal to mosquitoes and their larvae; it did much to diminish malaria in India and Ceylon after the First World War. Later, treatment of seed corn with DDT helped to increase the crop by killing the numerous ground insects which cause large losses.

In the 1950s many farmers reported an unusually high mortality of pigeons. The farmers were certainly not worried, because pigeons eat a great quantity of grain. Next came the more disturbing observation of a high death-rate among hawks. Hawks are birds of prey which feed on small mammals and birds. These smaller birds eat quantities of insects. Investigation showed that the small birds ingested DDT from the insects in amounts that were usually insufficient to cause death, but that the hawks obtained a more massive and fatal dose by eating a number of contaminated birds. The same thing happens to man; since DDT is persistent, people will absorb the unaltered pesticide by eating farm products which have been treated with it or have ingested it. Almost everyone in Europe and America now carries a certain amount of DDT in his body. In Britain the average is 2-3 parts per million, about one-hundredth of an ounce for an eleven-stone man. The average citizen of the United States carries nearly four times this amount. The former United Nations Secretary-General, U Thant, has estimated that about 1,000,000 pounds of DDT have been distributed over the world's surface since the Second World War. DDT and its derivatives are now the most widely spread synthetic chemicals on earth. DDT has been found in birds and fish of the Antarctic, thousands of miles from the nearest centre of dispersion. Lethal concentrations, such as were found in hawks, are rare, but there is disturbing evidence that sub-lethal concentrations may exert a pernicious long-term effect by reducing reproductive ability.

In July 1969 Professor Barry Commoner of Washington University, Missouri, sounded a grim warning. He said that, unless urgent action is taken, the fields and waters of North America will reach a point of no return within twenty-five to fifty years' time. Professor Commoner argued that pollution is largely due to avoidable faults of technology. Many other scientists have issued similar warnings.

There is some evidence that the products of combustion, the main pollutants of the air, may be a cause of cancers. In the middle years of the eighteenth century Percivall Pott, a London surgeon, described a type of cancer of the male genital organs which seemed to be confined to chimney-sweeps and workers whose clothing was persistently contaminated with sooty tars. Much the same type, this time of the lip, was commonly thought to be due to smoking clay pipes. Cancer of the tongue, more frequent in the nineteenth century than nowadays, may have been caused by heavy pipe smoking.

All tobacco smoke is a product of combustion. The smoker makes for himself a highly polluted but local atmosphere. If he ejects the smoke as soon as it enters his mouth, only a small proportion will reach his lungs. If he inhales the smoke, a large proportion will do so. The lungs must have accustomed themselves to a degree of pollution. But it does not necessarily follow that they will tolerate any higher degree of pollution. The evidence is clear that greatly increased pollution, whether by cigarette smoke or smog, is harmful. The dweller in a nineteenth-century industrial city may have escaped lung cancer because he did not create his own polluted atmosphere with cigarette smoke.

All authorities are agreed that most pollution is preventible, whether of air, water or soil. Attempts to reduce obvious pollution have been made from very early times. A Statute of 1273 prohibited the burning of sea-coal in London; a man was actually executed for committing this offence in 1306. But coal was too convenient a household fuel; London had become so smoky by the sixteenth century that Queen Elizabeth I found herself 'greatly grieved and annoyed with the taste and smoke of the sea-coals'. John Evelyn submitted a plan for smoke prevention to Charles II, and various attempts were made to diminish emission of smoke from factories in the nineteenth century. Almost the only practical effect of legislation was to ensure that smoke contaminated the air well above ground level by means of high chimneys. The smog episode of 1952 focused attention on the problem and directly instigated the Clean Air Act of 1956. But it is only the *visible* part of the smoke which has been reduced. The polluting gases, sulphur dioxide, carbon monoxide and carbon dioxide, and all the products of petrol and oil combustion, still flow into the atmosphere unchecked, the latter close to ground level. These pollutants probably do as much harm as the more obviously contaminating solid particles. One major advance is the decision of petrol companies not to treat petrol with lead salts. Lead pollution, caused almost entirely by the internal combustion engine, was rising dangerously.

Pollution can be very greatly reduced. It is possible to eliminate sulphur dioxide by washing, though the process is an expensive one and requires 35 tons of water for every ton of coal burned. There is no need to discharge untreated sewage into rivers. Factory effluents can be rendered innocuous. Short acting, selective pesticides are as effective as the persistent mass killer, DDT. There is no real necessity to use large quantities of freely soluble nitrogenous fertilizers on the land. Another form of pollution—excessive noise—is equally easily prevented. Long exposure to noise above 85 decibels can impair hearing; the risk is much greater above 95 decibels, which is the kind of noise level met in a boiler-shop. At 140 decibels (jet engines) a few minutes' exposure can cause severe permanent damage. Intermittent noise at lower decibel strengths may give rise to irritability, a feeling of fatigue and inability to perform skilled work. These gross manifestations are by no means the worst effects of noise. The roar of aeroplanes, the din of motor-cars and motor-bicycles, impair concentration and break sleep. The modern demand for sedatives and for drugs such as benzedrine, which help concentration in adverse conditions, is largely induced by a noisy environment. Yet noise pollution can be prevented. Adequate silencers will quieten any machine, but the engine is more expensive and not so efficient. It is, in fact, cheaper to impose a dangerous level of noise upon the public than to silence the machine, just as it is cheaper to permit efflux of noxious factory waste, to pour untreated sewage into rivers, to use long-lasting and mass-killing insecticides, to produce heavy crops with nitrogenous fertilizers. The problem is basically an economic one.

Another enormous problem is that of food and its distribution. Until quite recently, communities could starve when supplies of food were close at hand. Famine, one of our age-old enemies, was often local. In years of general plenty, the slow-moving ox-carts could carry grain from inland areas to the seaports, but beasts and drovers must be fed on the way. A regionally good harvest could not benefit those who lived at the centre of a destitute area. Low yields reduced agriculture to subsistence-farming, leaving only a small surplus to feed non-productive regions. The frequent mention of 'famine' is found throughout in monastic chronicles, the reference being to local scarcity rather than to general dearth. Widespread failure of crops might follow an adverse weather pattern. Famine then developed upon a national or continental scale. Such major disasters were probably comparatively uncommon, but the whole of Europe sometimes experienced acute general shortage; the years 1257-9 and 1346-7 are examples.

Better methods of farming slowly developed, culminating in the great agricultural reforms of the eighteenth century. Selective breeding of stock became possible with the introduction of clover, turnips and other winter feed. Chemical fertilizers such as guano reinforced animal manures. Potatoes, first introduced about 1580 into Spain from Peru, perhaps by way of Virginia, started to be grown as a field crop 200 years later. The corn harvest was vastly increased partly by good farming and partly by hybridization. The fourteenth-century farmer sowed $2\frac{1}{2}$ bushels or 157 pounds of wheat per acre and reaped a return of $7\frac{1}{2}$ bushels or $4\frac{1}{2}$ hundredweights. A twentieth-century farmer sows 3 bushels or 189 pounds and expects a return of about 2 tons. After making provision for next year's sowing, the fourteenth-century farmer had only twice the weight of his seed available as food. The modern farmer has twenty-two times the weight of seed available. More prolific bread corns, the possibility of maintaining beasts throughout the winter and new crops widened the margin which divided plenty from dearth.

Faster transport, first by metalled roads, then by canal barge, and later by railway, permitted carriage of bulky goods over long distances in a reasonable time. Local famine became an evil of the past but prolonged drought or incessant rainfall could still affect the national harvest and produce country-wide shortage. The Napoleonic wars brought advances in ship-building; larger and swifter vessels allowed import of corn in times of national dearth. The greatest change came when the new countries were able to feed the old. Ploughing of the vast prairie lands of North America, ranching of sheep and cattle in Australia, New Zealand, the United States and Argentina made available quantities of food over and above the local requirement.

Efficient means of preservation and rapid bulk transport allowed stockpiling against dearth and enabled non-producing countries to draw supplies from nations with an agricultural surplus. The margin between plenty and famine had widened to such an extent that no one who was able to pay for alien foodstuffs need ever go hungry. Preservation and increased mobility permitted survival and extension of the industrial city. The sprawling factory towns of the nineteenth century could never have been victualled by fourteenth-century farming and transport, when towns could only be fed because they were small and because the farmlands lay at their gates. The nineteenth-century city did not depend upon the farm, but drew supplies from the docks and railway goods-yard. Those supplies had their origin several thousand miles away. The small market town lost its importance and the industrial city became the centre of distribution. This shift produced the curious anomaly that the town worker ate a better diet than did the indigenous farm labourer who produced food.

Hunger remained, but hunger resulted from lack of purchasing power rather than from natural causes. Failure of the home harvest had little effect upon an importing nation. It needed two wars to point the moral that the bulk of Europe lives only by grace of the producing countries. Blockade and submarine warfare diminished supplies to a dangerously low level; starvation of the civilian population was deliberately used as a potent weapon. In 1915, British agriculture, undersold by cheap food imports, had sunk so low that it could only feed one-third of the population. Now, as the result of improved farming and the urgent need to establish a balance of payments, nearly half of Britain's food is home-produced.

Since Britain lives by exchanging manufactured goods for the remaining food she needs, a severe recession of trade or the refusal of exporting countries to send supplies could have a similar effect as a war, if upon a lesser scale. Britain would then be in the same position as an under-developed nation, for under-development implies the inability to make use of resources in order to ensure a reasonable standard of living. This is why there is still hunger, often approaching famine, in many parts of the world. An under-developed country cannot feed its excess population and cannot produce sufficient manufactured goods or raw materials to pay for imported food.

The inhabitants of under-developed countries are too often forced to live upon a subsistence agriculture, just as the European peoples of 1400 did. The farmer can produce sufficient food for his own family but has little to spare for non-productive members of the community. An African or Indian of today may be just as badly affected by local failure of the crop as was the fourteenth-century European. The Irish famines of 1846-9 and the pressures which followed resulted from failure of a subsistence agriculture. Ireland had a population of 8 million in 1800, almost entirely composed of peasants who supported themselves by cultivating a small rented acreage. In 1586-8 Sir Walter Raleigh introduced culture of the potato on his Irish estate of Youghal. The climate suited the large 'horse' potato which, by the end of the seventeenth century, had become a staple food. In 1800 the Irish peasantry, although poor and oppressed by alien landlords, were a healthy, well-fed nation. Potatoes and cabbage enabled them to rear pigs; they ate a good mixed diet of these vegetables, varied with small quantities of pork and dairy products. In 1845 potato disease, or blight, appeared locally; in 1846 virtually the entire potato crop was destroyed. The whole economy of Ireland collapsed in a few months. Within three years between 2 million and 3 million Irish died from starvation and famine sicknesses.

Landlords evicted hundreds of tenant families, their action dictated partly by greed for rent but also by a genuine belief that the country could be saved only through improvement of agriculture, impossible on the tiny under-capitalized holdings. In the distress which followed, over 1 million Irish emigrated to seek a new life in the British colonies or, more often, in the United States of America.

These were new lands, underpopulated, with a huge acreage of virgin soil awaiting the plough. They were good lands, better than the homeland which the emigrant had known. The nineteenth-century Irishman continued a tradition which has existed at least since the days of the Roman Empire and probably long before. Hunger and disease dictated the western movement of the Mongol hordes into Europe. A rising population and a scanty food supply urged Norsemen to pillage and colonize western Europe, to strike down through Russia, and on into modern Turkey.

The majority of the Irish emigrants found a better life in these young, under-developed countries. A modern Indian or African cannot do the same. There is little virgin territory of attractive quality remaining. It will require a huge expenditure of money and labour to bring the waterless deserts, the frozen wastes and the tropical forests into productive cultivation. Yet it must be done if man is to survive upon this planet for many years to come. More, the hitherto untapped sources of food must be brought under contribution by exploring the deep seas, by making use of the growth-power of algae, by finding unconventional sources of protein. An equable distribution of present supplies, less to developed and more to undeveloped countries, is certainly desirable now, but total production also needs to rise greatly if all people are to be well fed. India, most of Africa, parts of South America, and probably China are all undernourished. It has been said that world food production must rise by 170 per cent and protein foods such as meat and fish by five times the present amount during the next thirty years if these countries are to be properly fed and protein-deficiency diseases of the kwashiorkor type are to be ended.

The problem is urgent, far more urgent than the majority of people believe. The reason for this urgency is to be found in another difficulty which is entirely man-made. Man has opted out of the balanced antibiotic-symbiotic mechanism which provides a natural control of his increase. He once formed a part of this balance; he ate and was eaten. If the hunter encountered a deer and killed it, he ate well; if he encountered a sabre-toothed tiger, then the tiger ate well. All benefited all. The deer ate grass, man ate the deer, the tiger ate man and deer, the grass was nourished by the waste of man, deer and tiger. Species dwindled if they could not adapt themselves to this life; they flourished and became dominant because, through slow genetic changes, they were better able to fight or to escape, to eat or to avoid being eaten. Man developed a particular talent for using his hands and his brain. He started to reason and to communicate, to work with fire, stone, bronze and iron. Thus he was able to subdue enemies stronger than himself, to opt out of the natural rule of eat and be eaten.

Our remote forefathers died as do the majority of wild animals, from physical combat, from accident and from the process of aging. Disease as we know it today must have been rare except in so far as it formed part of terminal age. As men advanced and supported themselves by agriculture, the family increased to form the tribe, the village and the city. New enemies appeared with the birth of the crowd. Man defeated his larger enemies but, just as the African explorer had reason to fear the smaller creatures more than the greater, so the early civilizations soon encountered incursions of pestilence: infections of men, murrains which attacked their domesticated herds, blights which ruined their field-grown crops. These, in their turn, imposed a check upon rapid increase. By providing host bodies for a multitude of bacteria, man still formed part of a natural symbiotic-antibiotic balance.

We have seen something of the damping effect of disease upon exuberant growth in various chapters of this book. But it was not the great plagues, the Black Death, typhus fever and pandemics of cholera which had the most profound influence. The checks which the major disasters of sickness, famine and war imposed were only temporary. Chronic malnutrition played a greater part than acute starvation; the infectious ills of childhood and the hazards of childbirth killed far more people in the long term than did the more dramatic manifestations of epidemic disease. For thousands of years man had no knowledge of the cause and so no means of prevention or cure. He accepted that almost 250 out of every 1,000 children born must die within the first twelve months of life and that the average adult could not expect to live beyond the age of forty.

The middle years of the nineteenth century saw a change. This was only in part due to the discovery of bacteria and so to knowledge of the cause of many diseases. Prevention of lethal infections by inoculation, provision of sewerage and pure water, ample and cheaper supplies of food, a more humane attitude to suffering, all exerted a greater effect. The sum of these advances made for survival: population increased because more people survived for a longer time. But the beginnings of the European 'population explosion' antedated medical and social reform. It is difficult to explain the sudden expansion which occurred in the first half of the nineteenth century. During the 450 years from 1300 to 1750, the population of Europe rose from about 80 to 150 million; in the one century 1750-1850, another 115 million were added. Bubonic plague was the only great killer to disappear entirely from the European scene but the effect can hardly account for this large increase unless the mortality of plague has been wildly underestimated. The one obvious change in living conditions is from the rural village to the industrial town. Possibly the inevitable interbreeding of small, isolated communities led to loss of fertility. A wider range of people, drawn into the towns from many areas, and a lower age of marriage, may have removed a previous check to rising population.

Since 1850 the increase has approached the astronomical as a result of the general advances mentioned above. Mortality in the first year of life fell from nearly 160 per 1,000 live births in 1851 to 30 in 1951. In 1851 average life expectancy was 40 years, in 1921 57, and in 1951 67 years. By 1967 the average age of European males at death was 72. In 1850 the population of Europe stood at 265 million, in 1900 at 400, in 1950 at 550, while the present figure is in excess of 639 and probably nearer 650 million. American figures are masked by immigration during the past century but the population of the USA, which stood at just over 5 million in 1800, had risen to 31 million in 1850 and was over 180 million at the 1960 census. The figure for the census year 1970 is estimated to exceed 208 million. Taking the whole world, in which some areas like Africa and Asia still suffer a high infant mortality and low expectation of life, population has increased from 1,000 million in 1850 to 2,475 in 1950 and 3,570 million in 1970. Today there are almost four times as many people on earth as a hundred years ago.

Relaxation or leisure has combined with an uncontrolled rise in population and a high standard of living to produce another set of problems. The modern idea of 'a good life' demands and depends upon the amenities made available by technology. The automobile has added greatly to the comfort and enjoyment of life but has also imposed a number of formidable dangers. Noise and atmospheric pollution are but two. Whereas our remote ancestors sometimes encountered a sabre-toothed tiger when they left their caves in the morning, the modern commuter is more likely to meet his death in a motor-car accident. The sabre-toothed tiger at least benefited; the motor-car does not. Further, it is probable that the mortality directly attributable to motor traffic accidents is less than the indirect mortality imposed by the motor-car.

Increasing life span, overeating, oversmoking, the worries and stresses of modern life, have all contributed to a changed pattern of disease. If we take the middle-age group of 45-64, we find that accident of all kind produces an annual death rate of only 0.49 per 1,000 people. Cancer accounts for 3.25 deaths per 1,000. Arteriosclerotic heart disease or coronary thrombosis causes 2.31 deaths per 1,000 every year. There may be an association between exhaust pollution and cancer of the lung; the association between the motor-car and coronary thrombosis is equally probable. Overeating, worry and lack of exercise are the precipitating causes of this common form of death in middle age. The sedentary business man, who never walks when he can ride in a car, who eats and drinks and smokes too much, who spends his time in traffic jams worrying and fuming that he will be late for his next appointment, is the typical candidate for a 'coronary'. We can say with some certainty that he would be at far less risk if he simply left his car in the garage and walked.

The changed pattern of disease is due in part to changed habits of living, and in part to medical and para-medical advances. The great modern killers are the perils to which old people are exposed, the degenerative disorders of heart and blood-vessels, the chronic and acute respiratory illnesses, the cancers which seem to be part of the aging process. This type of disease annually accounts for 60 deaths per 1,000 of population in persons over 65 years old, while all other causes of death account for only 9 per 1,000. The total annual mortality is only 1.27 per 1,000 at age 15-44 and 10.45 per 1,000 at age 45-64. These figures show that the modern 'death pattern' is one of physical decay rather than of acute illness. It is entirely different from that which obtained 200 years ago. Infantile diarrhoea carried off thousands of babies in their first months of life; smallpox and measles destroyed children in their first decade; tuberculosis killed multitudes in their prime; sweeping pandemics of bubonic plague, typhus fever and cholera massacred their hundreds of thousands; typhoid and dysentery placed all age groups at risk. The control of these virulent infections has altered the pattern of death.

Control but not abolition. All these diseases still exist. Epidemics of some of them occur in developed countries but improved treatment has reduced mortality to a negligible figure. This is a very recent development. Until the Second World War absence of pandemics depended solely upon preventive and social medicine; if control had broken down and the pandemic occurred, doctors would have been as powerless to save life as their predecessors in the fourteenth century. Only since 1941 has the increasingly wide range of antibiotic drugs permitted attack upon the organism once it has invaded the human body. Control is not equally effective in all parts of the world. The pattern of disease in large areas, such as Africa, China and India, is broadly similar to that which obtained in Europe and North America a century ago. Cholera, typhus fever, smallpox, tuberculosis and malaria combine with malnutrition and squalid living conditions to cause a high infant mortality and to reduce expectation of life. The challenge of disease still remains.

The modern pattern of disease in developed countries results in a large increase of the older age group. There are at present reckoned to be about $19\frac{1}{2}$ million people aged 65 and over in the USA, and this figure will probably rise to nearly 25 million in 1985. If the average age of retirement from productive work remains at 65, then this large number of elderly people must be supported by the efforts of the younger. But this is not the whole story. The average age of starting productive work is 17 and there are at present about 74 million below this age; the estimated figure for 1985 is 106 million. The total population of the USA today is about 208 million and in 1985 will be 274 million. Thus today almost 94 million unproductive citizens must be supported by the efforts of 114 million productive ones and in 1985 the ratio will be 130 to 143 millions. Since life expectancy is rising, the problem may be a serious one by the year 2000. A century ago the 'useless mouths' were virtually confined to the lower age group; the task of supporting the elderly was almost negligible.

Lack of discipline lies at the root of all the troubles mentioned in this chapter. Man is conducting his life entirely for his own present benefit and with no thought for the morrow. Pollution, venereal disease, over-eating on one hand and hunger on the other, uncontrolled rise in population, where are these leading us and how can we avoid disaster? For disaster must be inevitable if we continue upon our present course. Man cannot pollute his surroundings to an unlimited degree without massive harm to himself. Man cannot breed unchecked without ultimately using up all sources of food supply on earth. The date upon which such an eventuality will arrive is problematical and we shall attempt no forecast here. But one thing is certain. That day will come, probably far sooner than we expect, unless we make urgent efforts to prevent or postpone its coming. Dr Norman Borlaug, awarded the 1970 Nobel Peace Prize for his work on developing improved strains of wheat, took the opportunity to urge the need for restriction of population growth. 'Without that,' he declared, 'our work will have been useless.'

There may, of course, be new worlds to conquer. Somewhere in space there must exist at least one habitable planet with an atmosphere, climatic conditions and a flora and fauna somewhat similar to our own. Such a planet could be colonized with our own foodstuffs and our own people. But, in order to keep world population static at its present figure, it would today be necessary to fire off 150,000 people into space every twenty-four hours. By the year 2000 population will be about double what it is today and will be increasing even more rapidly. We may find a habitable planet and we may be able to persuade a sufficient number of people to live on it, but we cannot stake our existence on the chance.

Lack of food is not the only danger. Diseases have been known to emerge from restricted areas in the past and they may emerge again, causing world-wide pandemics against which modern medicine will not necessarily prevail. Such viral diseases are known to exist. The Marburg virus, apparently transmitted by imported monkeys, killed seven of thirty-one victims in West Germany and Yugoslavia; the Machupo virus caused hundreds of deaths from haemorrhagic fever in Bolivia; in 1969 and 1970 an unidentified sickness struck the two townships of Lassa and Jos in Nigeria, bringing death to both natives and whites. The Lassa virus proved so lethal when investigated in the laboratories of Yale University that work upon it had to be stopped. Sheer pressure of numbers and of hunger may dictate a return to Mongolian and Viking type invasions; since all the more desirable parts of the world are now thickly inhabited, global war would inevitably result.

Disciplined human reproduction is the essential but not the only requirement. A fair distribution of food supplies is of equal urgency. Not so long ago, the wealthy members of a community ate luxuriously while the poorest classes starved. Today the differential is narrower at national level but has widened as between richer and poorer countries. A truly civilized nation no longer tolerates starvation among its underprivileged citizens; a truly civilized world would not accept the situation in which one half of its inhabitants ate too much while the other half ate too little. The difficulty of equable distribution, as of population control, largely arises from the concept of races and nationalities. If Man destroys himself, his destruction will most probably result from his obsessive emphasis upon the differences rather than the similarities between the races and nations. The primitive hates and fears are still with us, ready to break through the thin skins of civilization. Hate and fear cannot form a basis for the world-wide co-operation by which alone Man can save himself.

Medicine, social, therapeutic, and preventive, has given the human race opportunities for a longer and more healthy life. It has enabled the world population to expand. In doing so, it has brought problems which *may* be insoluble. Advancing technology has given us comforts and amenities undreamed of two centuries ago. In doing so, it has brought problems which also *may* be insoluble. The combination of the two has caused Man, in material things, to run ahead of his own state of civilization. The primitive is not buried deeply enough for safety. This is why Man lives basically like an animal, breeding unchecked, fouling his surroundings, exhausting his resources, taking no thought for the future. Governments tell us that 'we must come to terms with our environment', but this is begging the question. Man must come to terms with himself. If he does not learn self-discipline, if he fails to solve the problems which he has created, then, at least temporarily, those problems will be solved for him. The solution will lie in the hands of one or all of his age-old enemies, Famine, Pestilence and War, the Three Horsemen of the Apocalypse, who bring in their train the Fourth Rider, Death upon his Pale Horse.

Bibliography

General

ADAMS, F., *The Genuine Works of Hippocrates*, Sydenham Society, London, 1849. (revised) Williams and Wilkins, Baltimore, 1939.

BETT, W. R., *The History and Conquest of Common Diseases*, University of Oklahoma Press, Norman, 1954.

GALE, A. H., *Epidemic Diseases*, Penguin, Harmondsworth, 1959. (pb.)

HENSCHEN, F., *The History of Diseases*, Longmans, London, 1966.

L'ETANG, H., *The Pathology of Leadership*, Heinemann, London, 1969.

SCOTT, H. H., *Some Notable Epidemics*, Arnold, London, 1934.

SCOTT STEVENSON, R., *Famous Illnesses in History*, Eyre and Spottiswoode, London, 1962.

SHREWSBURY, J. F. D., *The Plague of the Philistines*, Gollancz, London, 1964.

YEARSLEY, M., *Le Roy est Mort*, Unicorn Press, London, 1935.

Chapter One

ALLBUTT, SIR T. C., *Greek Medicine in Rome*, Macmillan, London, 1921.
CHADWICK, H., *The Early Church*, Penguin, Harmondsworth, 1967. (pb.)
CLAY, R. M., *The Mediaeval Hospitals of England*, Methuen, London, 1909.
CRAWFURD, R., *Plague and Pestilence in Literature and Art*, Clarendon Press, Oxford, 1914.
JONES, A. H. M., *The Later Roman Empire*, 3 vols. Blackwell, Oxford, 1964.
PROCOPIUS, *The Persian War*, Loeb Classical Library, Heinemann, London, 1914.
SCHOUTEN, J., *The Rod and Serpent of Asklepios*, Elsevier, Amsterdam, 1967.

Chapter Two

BELL, W. G., *The Great Plague in London in 1665*, John Lane, London, 1924.
COHN, N., *The Pursuit of the Millenium*, Secker & Warburg, London, 1957. Paladin, London, 1970. (pb.)
CREIGHTON, C., *A History of Epidemics in Britain*, 2 vols. Cambridge University Press, 1891.
GOODRIDGE, J. F., *Langland, Piers the Ploughman*, Penguin, Harmondsworth, 1959. (pb.)
SHREWSBURY, J. F. D., *A History of Bubonic Plague in the British Isles*, Cambridge University Press, 1970.
(Shrewsbury's conclusions should not be accepted without consulting Morris, C., *The Plague in Britain*, Historical Journal, vol. xiv, No. 1. March 1971.)
SOUTHERN, R. W., *The Mediaeval Church*, Penguin, Harmondsworth, 1970. (pb.)
ZIEGLER, P., *The Black Death*, Collins, London, 1969. Penguin, Harmondsworth, 1970. (pb.)

Chapter Three

CHAPMAN, H. W., *The Last Tudor King*, Jonathan Cape, London, 1958. Arrow Books, London, 1961. (pb.)
ELTON, G. R., *England Under the Tudors*, Methuen, London, 1955.
GOODMAN, H., *Contributors to the Knowledge of Syphilis*, Froben, New York, 1944.
GRAHAM, STEPHEN, *Ivan the Terrible*, Ernest Benn, London, 1932.
HOLCOMBE, R. C., *Who Gave the World Syphilis?*, Froben, New York, 1937.
HUDSON, E. H., *Trepanematosis*, Oxford University Press, 1946.
—— *Non-Venereal Syphilis*, Livingstone, Edinburgh, 1958.
MACLAURIN, C., *Post Mortem*, Jonathan Cape, London, 1923.
MACNALTY, SIR A., *Henry VIII: A Difficult Patient*, Christopher Johnson, London, und.
SCARISBRICK, J. J., *Henry VIII*, Eyre and Spottiswoode, London, 1968. Penguin, Harmondsworth, 1971. (pb.)
UDEN, G., *They Looked Like This*, Blackwell, Oxford, 1965.

Chapter Four

HEROLD, J. C., *The Age of Napoleon*, Weidenfeld and Nicolson, London, 1964. Penguin, Harmondsworth, 1969. (pb.)

KEMBLE, J., *Napoleon Immortal*, John Murray, London, 1959.

MARKHAM, F., *Napoleon*, Weidenfeld and Nicolson, London, 1963. Mentor, London, 1966. (pb.)

PRINZIG, F., *Epidemics Resulting from Wars*, Clarendon Press, Oxford, 1916.

ZINSSER, H., *Rats, Lice, and History*, George Routledge, London (4th Ed.), 1942.

Chapter Five

ELLIOTT, J. H., *The Old World and the New 1492-1650*, Cambridge University Press, 1970.

GREENHILL, W. A., *Rhazes on Small-pox and Measles*, Sydenham Society, London, 1848.

PARRY, J. H., *The Spanish Seaborne Empire*, Hutchinson, London, 1966.

PRESCOTT, W. H., *History of the Conquest of Mexico*, Bentley, London, 1843.

ROLLESTON, J. D., *The History of the Acute Exanthemata*, Heinemann, London, 1937.

Chapter Six

BROCKINGTON, C. F., *A Short History of Public Health*, Churchill, London (2nd Ed.), 1966.

CURTIN, P. D., *The Image of Africa: British Ideas and Action 1780-1850*, University of Wisconsin Press, Madison, 1964.

FOSTER, W. D., *A History of Parasitology*, Livingstone, Edinburgh, 1965.

GELFAND, M., *Livingstone the Doctor*, Blackwell, Oxford, 1957.

HAGGARD, H. W., *Devils, Drugs and Doctors*, Heinemann, London, 1929.

JARAMILLO-ARANGO, J., *The Conquest of Malaria*, Heinemann, London, 1950.

SNOW, J., *On Cholera* (Reprint), Hafner, New York, 1965.

Chapter Seven

CARTER, C. O., *Human Heredity*, Penguin, Harmondsworth, 1962. (pb.)

MACALPINE, I., and HUNTER, R., *George III and the Mad Business*, Allen Lane, London, 1969.

—— *Porphyria, a Royal Malady*, B.M.A., London, 1968.

MASSIE, R. K., *Nicholas and Alexandra*, Gollancz, London, 1968. Pan Books, London, 1969. (pb.)

PARES, SIR B., *The Fall of the Russian Monarchy*, Cape, London, 1939.

SETON WATSON, H., *The Decline of Imperial Russia*, Methuen, London, 1952. University Paperbacks, 1964.

TAYLOR, E., *The Fossil Monarchies*, Weidenfeld and Nicolson, London, 1963. Penguin, Harmondsworth, 1967. (pb.)

WILSON, C., *Rasputin*, Arthur Barker, London, 1964. Panther Books, London, 1966. (pb.)
YOUSSOUPOFF (Prince), *Rasputin*, Jonathan Cape, London, 1927.

Chapter Eight

BRACHER, K., *The German Dictatorship*, Weidenfeld and Nicolson, London, 1971.
BULLOCK, A., *Hitler, a Study in Tyranny*, Odhams, London, 1952. Penguin, Harmondsworth, 1962. (pb.)
COHN, N., *Warrant for Genocide*, Eyre and Spottiswoode, London, 1967. Penguin, Harmondsworth, 1970. (pb.)
PERNOUD, R., *Joan of Arc by Herself and Her Witnesses*, Macdonald, London, 1964. Penguin, Harmondsworth, 1969. (pb.)
THOMAS, K., *Religion and the Decline of Magic*, Weidenfeld and Nicolson, London, 1971.
TREVOR-ROPER, H., *The European Witch-Craze of the 16th and 17th Centuries*, Penguin, Harmondsworth, 1969. (pb.)

Chapter Nine

BRIERLEY, J. K., *Biology and the Social Crisis*, Heinemann, London, 1967.
CIPOLLA, C. M., *The Economic History of World Population*, Penguin, Harmondsworth, 1962. (pb.)

Index of Names

Index of Subjects